ULTRA SIMPLE

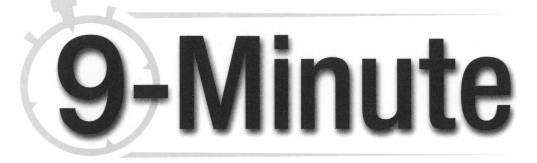

9-Minute Workouts

By Alex A. Lluch
Health and Fitness Expert &
Author of Over 4 Million Books Sold!

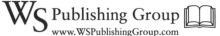

WS Publishing Group
www.WSPublishingGroup.com
San Diego, California

Ultra Simple 9-Minute Workouts

By Alex A. Lluch

Nutritional and fitness guidelines based on information provided by the United States Food and Drug Administration, Food and Nutrition Information Center, National Agricultural Library, Agricultural Research Service, and the U.S. Department of Agriculture.

For more best-selling titles by WS Publishing Group,
visit www.wspublishinggroup.com.

Exercise Photos:
Nathaniel Kam, www.nathanielkamphotography.com

Model:
Anicka Pantano, ZARZAR Models, www.zarzarmodels.com
Leonardo Cerqueira, www.modelmayhem.com/1013282

Printed in China

ISBN 13: 978-1-936061-39-6

DISCLAIMER: The content in this book is provided for general informational purposes only and is not meant to substitute the advice provided by a medical professional. This information is not intended to diagnose or treat medical problems or substitute for appropriate medical care. If you are under the care of a physician and/or take medications for diabetes, heart disease, hypertension, or any other condition, consult your health-care provider prior to initiation of any dietary program. Implementation of a dietary program may require altercation in your medication needs and must be done by or under the direction of your physician. If you have or suspect that you have a medical problem, promptly contact your health-care provider. Never disregard professional medical advice or delay in seeking it because of something you have read in this book.

WS Publishing Group, Inc. makes no claims whatsoever regarding the interpretation or utilization of any information contained herein and/or recorded by the user of this journal. If you utilize any information provided in this book, you do so at your own risk and you specifically waive any right to make any claim against the author and publisher, its officers, directors, employees, or representatives as the result of the use of such information. Consult your physician before making any changes in your diet or exercise.

contents

> **"** The great thing in the world is not so much where we stand, as in what direction we are moving. **"**
>
> ~ Oliver Wendell Holmes

Introduction

Decades of research have proven that fitness and eating right are the greatest preventative measures for aging, disease, and early death. People who get regular exercise — even just minutes a day — feel better, live longer, and have more energy and confidence. And yet, 50 million Americans still live completely sedentary lives, meaning that they have desk-jobs, no regular physical activity program, and are generally inactive around the house or yard.

As a result, the U.S. is one of the fattest nations in the world, with 67 percent of Americans considered to be overweight, and 34 percent considered to be obese. Millions are struggling with their weight every day and suffering the effects, from lack of energy to infertility to diabetes to heart disease.

That's because so many exercise programs are doomed to fail. Not everyone who wants to get in shape has time for or is physically able to embark on an intense, time-consuming fitness regiment. It's just too easy to get overwhelmed and frustrated, and quit. That's why *Ultra Simple 9-Minute*

Workouts is such an effective program for getting fit, improving energy, and losing weight. Six days a week (the seventh day is for rest), you will perform two 9-minute workout plans, one in the morning and one in the evening, that combine either a cardio and upper body set, or a core and lower body set. With dozens of different combinations and multiple levels of difficulty, you'll never get bored or stagnant during this 9-week exercise program.

In just a few short minutes a day, you will exponentially improve your energy and mood while slimming down. Exercise will seamlessly become part of your everyday life, instead of feeling like a burden or chore. Forget slaving away at the gym or trying to find time for a 60-minute workout video, because *Ultra Simple 9-Minute Workouts* is designed for any fitness level, schedule, lifestyle, and age.

Getting in shape and losing weight are never easy. As we age and our metabolisms slow down, the body gets comfortable with the extra pounds and settles into a more sedentary lifestyle. Your body is like a car with a stalled battery, and *Ultra Simple 9-Minute Workouts* is the jump-start it needs!

How to Use This Book

Congratulations! You've taken the first step toward getting in shape and losing weight without even trying! Just 9 minutes, twice a day, 6 days a week and you'll be burning calories, increasing your energy, and toning your entire body. Really, what you're doing is changing your life for the better.

You'll find that this exercise program is not only ultra-effective, it's fun and never dull. You will be able to track your progress over the course of the 9 weeks and watch your body getting slimmer and stronger.

Ultra Simple 9-Minute Workouts offers many valuable features, including:

Your Personal Profile

Before you begin the *Ultra Simple 9-Minute Workouts*, you need to build your personal health and fitness profile. This section helps you assess your current physical state, habits, and preferences for diet and exercise. With this information, you will be able to determine where you started and how far you've come, as well as identify your goals and any potential obstacles.

Your Current Fitness Level

Before starting this exercise plan, you will want to assess your current fitness level in terms of heart rate, blood pressure, body composition, strength, and flexibility.

Calculating your BMI and other levels will give you an idea of whether or not your health status is putting you at risk for heart disease and other issues. If you are at risk, sticking to this exercise plan for 9 weeks will greatly improve your health. Research has shown that losing just 5 to 10 percent of your body weight can significantly improve a person's health by lowering cholesterol and the risk of heart disease, stroke, and diabetes.

The physical assessments in this chapter, including a push-up, sit-up, sit and reach, and squat test, will not only let you know how you stack up against the averages for your age and gender, but will also tell you what areas you can improve in.

At the end of this program, you will be amazed at how much improvement you've made!

9-Minute Exercises

Ultra Simple 9-Minute Workouts includes 72 unique exercises that, when combined, work the entire body, including the core, shoulders, back, arms, glutes, legs, and even the heart.

Monday through Saturday you will combine either 3 cardiovascular exercises in the morning with 3 exercises that work the upper body in the evening, or 3 exercises that work the core in the morning with 3 exercises that work the lower body in the evening. Sunday is your day to rest and recuperate.

The 9-Minute Exercises chapter includes full-color photos demonstrating each exercise, as well as complete instructions on how to properly perform the moves. Use this section to learn the correct technique and form for each exercise in the program.

Each day is divided into a morning and night set of exercises. You will perform each exercise in the set 3 times for 50 seconds, with 10 seconds of rest before moving on to the next exercise. By the time you have completed your 3 rounds of each exercise, your 9-minute workout will be finished! Simple and stress-free!

Additionally, the complete workout program is broken up into 3 levels of difficulty, with 3 weeks at each stage. As you get stronger and develop more stamina during the program, the exercises will get progressively more challenging. Don't be afraid of the challenge, because the harder you work, the more results you will see in less time.

Warming Up and Cooling Down

Always take a few minutes to stretch to prepare your muscles and prevent injury. Be sure to stretch before and after each of your 9-minute workouts.

Important stretches include holding the heel close to the glute to stretch the quad, reaching toward the toes to stretch hamstrings, calf stretches against a wall, and stretching your arms behind your head and across the chest to loosen shoulders, chest, biceps, and triceps.

Daily 9-Minute Workout Guide

Your daily workout guide shows the 3 exercises you will be performing in the morning and evening for each day. There is also a place to record the reps you are able to complete in each set. Writing down your reps for each set is a great way to compare and track your progress as you build strength and stamina.

The daily guide includes small photos of each exercise. You should refer back to the 9-Minute Exercises chapter to see step-by-step instructions and proper form for each exercise.

Motivational Stickers

Each daily workout guide page includes space to place an "I Did It!" sticker to help you keep track of the days when you complete your workout and meet your goals. Seeing the stickers on each page will give you motivation during the times when you feel like avoiding a set of exercises or skipping a day all together.

Your Personal Profile

Begin your workout program by gathering some information to assess your current physical state, habits, and preferences.

Fill in the information on the following pages. Visit your primary care physician and have your cholesterol, triglycerides, and blood pressure measured. These levels will also factor into the choices you make when creating your diet and fitness plan. You should also take your current measurements and place a "Before" photo in this section. It will be motivating to look back and see a visual of where you began and how far you have come.

Next, assess your diet and fitness history. You will also answer some questions about your past attempts to get in shape, and the obstacles you encountered. Finally, outline your goals. Determine what you hope to accomplish with this program, which types of physical activities you most enjoy, and more.

Good luck meeting all your goals!

Your Health Profile

Complete the following personal health profile. You can request necessary information from your primary health-care provider.

Name: _____   Triglycerides: _____

Age: _____   HDL Cholesterol: _____

Height: _____   LDL Cholesterol: _____

Total Cholesterol: _____   Blood Pressure: _____

Current Physical Activity: (sedentary, moderately active, very active)

_____

_____

_____

_____

Current Diet & Eating Habits: (fast food, snack often, late-night eating, etc.)

_____

_____

_____

Other Current Habits: (smoking, drinking, lack of sleep, etc.)

_____

_____

_____

_____

_____

_____

Dietary Habits Questionnaire

The following questions will assist you in developing your weight-loss program.

Which best describes your daily eating habits?
- ❑ 3 average meals
- ❑ Graze frequently
- ❑ 1 large meal, little else

What types of food do you crave the most?
- ❑ Meat/fish
- ❑ Fruit/vegetables
- ❑ Bread/cereals/rice
- ❑ Sweets

Do you typically eat out or prepare food for yourself?
- ❑ I usually cook my food
- ❑ I eat out or have pre-made meals

What is your weight-loss goal?
- ❑ Lose 10 or more pounds
- ❑ Maintain weight
- ❑ Lose a little weight
- ❑ Improve health

Which habits do you have?
- ❑ Skipping meals
- ❑ Drinking full-sugar soda
- ❑ Carb addiction
- ❑ Overeating while dining out

Describe your body type:
- ❑ Overweight
- ❑ Average
- ❑ Muscular

For what particular event (if any) do you want to lose weight?

_____

_____

_____

_____

_____

_____

_____

What is your number one reason for wanting to lose weight?

_____

_____

_____

_____

_____

Your Fitness History

It is important to look back at your past fitness experiences to determine the diet and workout plan that will have the greatest chance for success for you.

Is there any reason why you should not engage in physical activity?

_____

At what age were you in your best physical shape?

_____

Have you ever participated in a workout program? When?

_____

How long did you stay with the program?

_____

What did the program include?

_____

What led you to or inspired you to get into shape now?

_____

What obstacles have kept you from meeting your fitness goals?

_____

What will ensure these obstacles do not inhibit you this time?

_____

Rate your current fitness level on a scale of 1-10 (1=Worst 10=Best).

_____

Your Fitness Goals

By first identifying your goals, you can create a specific workout routine to help you achieve them. Your goals should be specific, quantifiable, realistic, and time-based. Fill out the following questions honestly and with a critical eye. You'll be able to use the resulting information to get inspired and ward off possible pitfalls.

What do you want to accomplish with your workout program?
(Check the boxes next to the goals that are most important to you.)

❑ Improve cardiovascular fitness and endurance

❑ Improve diet and/or eating habits

❑ Improve flexibility

❑ Improve health

❑ Improve strength

❑ Improve muscle tone and shape

❑ Increase energy

❑ Lose weight

❑ Prevent injury and/or rehabilitate injury

❑ Train for a sports-specific event

❑ Reduce cholesterol

❑ Reduce blood pressure

❑ Reduce risk of disease

❑ Reduce stress

❑ Gain weight

❑ Other: _____

❑ Other: _____

What types of physical activity do you like and dislike?

_____

_____

_____

_____

Do you prefer to exercise alone, with a partner, or in a group?

_____

_____

_____

_____

DATE:_____ WEIGHT:_____ BODY FAT %:_____

MEASUREMENTS:

[   ] chest   [   ] biceps   [   ] waist   [   ] hips   [   ] thighs

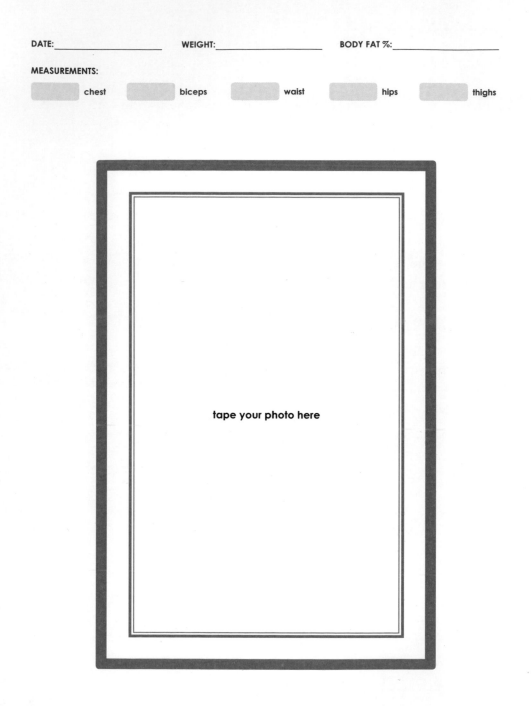

tape your photo here

PHOTO COMMENTS: _____

Your Current Fitness Level

Every individual has his or her unique potential for physical fitness based on the interaction of genetics, health status, and lifestyle. Therefore, the first step in getting fit is determining your current physical condition. This chapter contains a series of simple tests used to quantify your starting point on the road to fitness. You will be able to determine your risk for disease and where your fitness level falls in comparison to the average fit American. These statistics will help you prepare realistic goals and track personal progress and success. Once your new fitness plan is well underway, you can look back at these tables and see how you have improved in all areas.

Important reminder: A doctor should be consulted before beginning any rigorous exercise program. This is especially important if you are taking medication for high blood pressure or are being treated for any other physical condition, such as diabetes.

Assessing your current fitness level

Begin by assessing your current fitness level. Use this assessment to create a realistic fitness plan. This baseline assessment includes attention to:

❶ Heart rate
❷ Blood pressure
❸ Body composition
❹ Strength
❺ Flexibility

❶ Heart Rate

Heart rate is a leading indicator of your baseline fitness level and can be used as a guide to maximize the results of cardiovascular exercise. The heart is a specialized muscle that is designed to pump the blood needed to maintain all of your bodily functions. Blood brings oxygen and nutrients to every part of the body. A heart's performance is essential to sustaining life all the way down to the cellular level.

Your heart rate is the number of times your heart beats in a minute. This number is a clear indicator of the strength of your heart. A strong heart pumps more effectively with each contraction, and therefore doesn't need to beat as fast to supply the body with blood. A high heart rate indicates that the heart is not as efficient at circulating blood, and therefore needs to pump faster to keep up with your body's needs. As your heart becomes better at pumping blood through regular exercise, you will find that your heart rate will decrease. Find your resting and active heart rates. Use these numbers to determine your current fitness level.

A resting heart rate is simply the number of times the heart beats in a minute when you're not moving around. It is important that you sit or lie down and remain motionless for at least 2 minutes before taking this measurement. Once you're completely relaxed, place 2 fingers against the inside of the wrist or alongside the neck. Count the number of beats for 15 seconds and then multiply that number by 4.

An active heart rate indicates your heart's maximum potential or ability to work under strain. You can measure your active heart rate during exercise by purchasing a heart rate monitor. Also, many treadmills, ellipticals, and other fitness equipment will measure your active heart rate for you. Active heart rate is important for measuring improvement in your fitness level, specifically with regard to aerobic fitness.

Compare your heart rate to the table, which provides heart rate fitness levels by age and gender.

Resting Heart Rate Fitness by Age and Gender

MEN BY AGE GROUP

RESTING HEART RATE	AGE IN YEARS					
	18–25	26–35	36–45	46–55	56–65	65+
EXCELLENT	50–60	50–61	51–62	51–63	52–61	51–61
GOOD	61–68	62–69	63–69	64–70	62–70	62–68
AVERAGE	69–76	70–77	70–78	71–79	71–78	69–75
FAIR	77-80	78-80	79-81	80-83	79-80	76-78
POOR	81+	81+	82+	84+	81+	79+

WOMEN BY AGE GROUP

RESTING HEART RATE	AGE IN YEARS					
	18–25	26–35	36–45	46–55	56–65	65+
EXCELLENT	55–64	55–63	55–63	55–64	55–63	55–63
GOOD	65–72	64–71	64–72	65–72	64–72	64–71
AVERAGE	73–80	72–78	73–80	73–79	73–79	72–79
FAIR	81-83	79-81	81-83	80-82	80-82	80-81
POOR	84+	82+	84+	83+	83+	82+

❷ Blood Pressure

It is important to determine your blood pressure before starting a physical fitness program. Those suffering from high blood pressure should contact a medical professional before beginning any physical fitness routine. Blood pressure is the force of blood against the arteries, and is created by the heart as it pumps blood through the circulatory system. Like all muscles, the heart cycles between contracting and relaxing; blood pressure varies accordingly. Systolic blood pressure refers to the pressure when the heart contracts. Diastolic pressure refers to the pressure when the heart relaxes. Blood pressure is expressed by these two figures, with the systolic reading listed over the diastolic figure (e.g., 130/90).

Many pharmacies are equipped with machines that allow customers to measure their own blood pressure. This may serve as a quick way to generally measure baseline blood pressure, but your doctor can give you the most reliable reading. Compare your blood pressure to the table below, which lists blood pressure figures and their corresponding risk categories.

Blood Pressure and Corresponding Risk Level

SYSTOLIC	DIASTOLIC	STAGE AND HEALTH RISK
210	120	High Blood Pressure • Hypertension Stage 4 • Very Severe Risk
180	110	High Blood Pressure • Hypertension Stage 3 • Severe
160	100	High Blood Pressure • Hypertension Stage 2 • Moderate Risk
140	90	High Blood Pressure • Hypertension Stage 1 • Mild Risk
140	90	Borderline High
130	90	High Normal
120	85	Normal • Optimum
110	75	Low Normal
90	60	Borderline Low
60	40	Low Blood Pressure • Hypotension
50	33	Very Low Blood Pressure • Extreme Danger

Individuals who are overweight often suffer from high blood pressure, or hypertension. Hypertension is dangerous because it strains the heart as it pumps blood through the body. Over time, the strain can lead to heart muscle breakdown and deterioration. This leaves the heart weakened and increases the chance of a heart attack, stroke, and heart failure. In addition, hypertension can lead to chronic kidney failure.

❸ Body Composition

The body functions best when it consists of a proper proportion of muscle, fat, organs, and bone. Your body composition is determined by the ratio of these elements against the body's mass. While bone and organ mass and weight remain relatively constant, everyone's fat and muscle weight varies. The percent of body weight that is made up of fat and muscle is an important indicator of body composition and overall fitness. Without proper amounts of both muscle and fat, the body will fail to work at its optimum level.

A person who appears thin may still have a high fat percentage and therefore be unhealthy. People who undergo crash or extreme diets will often lose more muscle mass than fat. If you try to lose weight by dieting without exercising, lean muscle mass may decrease, resulting in an increased fat percentage. Exercise will keep that from happening. Regular exercise forces muscles to engage and work to exhaustion. This, coupled with adequate rest, forces your muscles to adapt by growing larger and stronger. The increased muscle mass diminishes your body's fat percentage and increases its overall health.

Fat is essential to many functions of the body. However, excess fat, especially in the waist area, puts you at increased risk of cardiovascular disease and other health problems such as heart attacks, strokes, and diabetes. In addition, new research shows a correlation between most forms of cancer (except skin cancer) and excess body fat. While genetic predispositions and environmental factors can put you at risk of developing cancer and many other diseases, excess weight increases these risks by making it more difficult for the body to fight off infection and rebuild damaged tissues.

Body composition and fat percentages can be determined in numerous ways:

Hydrostatic Weighing: The most accurate method of measuring body composition is called hydrostatic weighing. This involves weighing a person in air, and then again while submerged in water. However accurate this method might be, it is not very practical due to the specialized equipment needed and the complexity of the procedure.

Bioelectrical Impedance Analysis (BIA): The BIA is a computerized examination that helps medical professionals determine the specific composition of the body, including its fat percentage. This is a noninvasive test administered by a doctor and takes about 10 minutes. A BIA can also detect the presence of disease, nutrient and water deficiency, environmental and industrial pollutants, oxidative damage, and other ailments. With this information, a health-care provider can create a fitness and diet routine that helps correct a variety of conditions.

Caliper Test: The most common and relatively accurate method for measuring body fat is what's known as a skin fold, or caliper test. Using a specialized instrument called a caliper, the person conducting the test pinches folds of skin on various locations throughout the body. This test is available at many gyms or fitness facilities.

Body Mass Index (BMI): Less accurate than hydrostatic weighing or a caliper test, the BMI uses a person's height and weight to determine an approximate fat percentage. Health-care professionals often use a person's BMI to determine his or her cardiovascular health risk. While all bodies are different, they all generally conform to this scale. Although each person's frame varies, the range provided in the BMI takes this into consideration. Your BMI can be determined by taking your weight (in kilograms) and dividing it by its height (in meters) squared; the formula is simple: $Kg/m2$ = BMI. Your approximate BMI can be found using your body's height (feet) and weight (lbs) in the following table. This table also shows the cardiovascular risks associated with various ranges of BMI readings.

BMI and Cardiovascular Risk Chart for Men and Women

BMI	19	20	21	22	23	24	25	26	27	28	29	30	31	32	33	34	35
Height						Weight in pounds											
4'10"	91	96	100	105	110	115	119	124	129	134	138	143	148	153	158	162	167
4'11"	94	99	104	109	114	119	124	128	133	138	143	148	153	158	163	168	173
5'	97	102	107	112	118	123	128	133	138	143	148	153	158	163	158	174	179
5'1"	100	106	111	116	122	127	132	137	143	148	153	158	164	169	174	180	185
5'2"	104	109	115	120	126	131	136	142	147	153	158	164	169	175	180	186	191
5'3"	107	113	118	124	130	135	141	146	152	158	163	169	175	180	186	191	197
5'4"	110	116	122	128	134	140	145	151	157	163	169	174	180	186	192	197	204
5'5"	114	120	126	132	138	144	150	156	162	168	174	180	186	192	198	204	210
5'6"	118	124	130	136	142	148	155	161	167	173	179	186	192	198	204	210	216
5'7"	121	127	134	140	146	153	159	166	172	178	185	191	198	204	211	217	223
5'8"	125	131	138	144	151	158	164	171	177	184	190	197	203	210	216	223	230
5'9"	128	135	142	149	155	162	169	176	182	189	196	203	209	216	223	230	236
5'10"	132	139	146	153	160	167	174	181	188	195	202	209	216	222	229	236	243
5'11"	136	143	150	157	165	172	179	186	193	200	208	215	222	229	236	243	250
6'	140	147	154	162	169	177	184	191	199	206	213	221	228	235	242	250	258
6'1"	144	151	159	166	174	182	189	197	204	212	219	227	235	242	250	257	265
6'2"	148	155	163	171	179	186	194	202	210	218	225	233	241	249	256	264	272
6'3"	152	160	168	176	184	192	200	208	216	224	232	240	248	256	264	272	279
	Healthy					Overweight						Obese					

❹ Strength

Your body's physical strength shows the condition of your muscles and their ability to function at maximum output. Strength is the amount of force a muscle can produce. It can be measured in the amount of weight the muscle can lift or how much force it can exert as you jump, hit a golf ball, or engage in other activities. By measuring your muscles' strength, you can get a sense of your overall fitness. This measurement will help you create a fitness plan and measure future successes.

Push-up Test: This test focuses on the strength and endurance of muscles in your upper body. Gently stretch and warm up your arm, chest, and shoulder muscles. Avoid over-exertion in order to get the most accurate test results. Men should assume the traditional push-up position, with only the hands and tips of the toes touching the ground. Women should assume the bent knee position, with knees and hands touching the ground. No matter which position you use, you should keep the head, neck and back aligned. Start by bending your arms and slowly lowering your chest until it's 4 inches from the ground, keeping your back and legs straight. Then straighten the arms and push your body back into the starting position. Be sure not to lock your elbows. The back and legs should remain straight with the head and neck in line at all times. Repeat this as many times as you can while maintaining proper form. Count the number of repetitions before fatigue forces you to stop.

The following table will help you estimate your fitness level based on your age, gender, and the number of push-ups you can do.

Push-up Fitness for Men

	MEN'S AGE					
	13-19	20s	30s	40s	50s	60s
Excellent	45+	40+	35+	29+	25+	23+
Good	31-41	26-35	22-29	18-25	15-22	14-20
Average	26-29	22-25	18-21	15-17	12-14	10-13
Fair	14-24	12-21	9-17	7-14	5-11	3-9
Poor	14-	12-	9-	7-	5-	3-

Push-up Fitness for Women

	WOMEN'S AGE					
	13-19	20s	30s	40s	50s	60s
Excellent	32+	30+	28+	24+	20+	18+
Good	21–28	19–26	18–26	15–22	12–18	11–16
Average	17–20	16–18	14–17	12–14	10–12	8–10
Fair	9–16	8–15	5–13	4–11	3–9	2–7
Poor	8-	7-	4-	3-	2-	1-

NO. OF PUSH-UPS

Sit-Up Test: The sit-up test assesses your abdominal muscles' fitness and stamina. Lie on the floor, facing up with knees bent and place your feet shoulder-width apart. Start by pressing your lower back into the ground and place your arms across your chest. Lift your head, neck, and shoulders off the floor and bring your body into a sitting position by engaging the stomach muscles. The abdomen should be contracted as your upper body is brought to a 90-degree angle with the floor. Then slowly roll back down into the starting position while keeping the abdominal muscles tight.

Compare your number with the following chart.

1 Minute Sit-up Test for Men

	MEN'S AGE					
	18-25	26-35	36-45	46-55	56-65	65+
Excellent	49+	46+	42+	36+	32+	29+
Good	41–48	39–45	34–41	27-35	23–31	20–28
Average	34–40	31–38	25-33	21-26	16–22	14-19
Fair	30-33	29-30	22-24	18-20	14-15	11-13
Poor	29-	28-	21-	17-	13-	10-

1 Minute Sit-up Test for Women

	WOMEN'S AGE					
	18-25	26-35	36-45	46-55	56-65	65+
Excellent	43+	39+	33+	27+	24+	23+
Good	35–42	31–38	25–32	20–26	16–23	15–22
Average	28–34	24–30	18–24	13–19	9–15	10–14
Fair	23–27	19–23	14–17	9–12	6–8	4–9
Poor	22-	18-	13-	8-	5-	3-

Squat Test: The Squat Test focuses on the strength of the lower body. Stand up straight with your feet shoulder-width apart. Just as if you are sitting back into a chair, bring your hips back, and lower your body until your upper legs are parallel to the floor. Keep your knees and heels aligned at all times. With your head and chest lifted, return to a standing position. A chair may be placed underneath as a guide, but must not be used to rest in between squats. Count how many squats are completed before you tire and must stop.

Compare your number with the following chart.

Squats Fitness Determined by Age

		AGE				
		18-25	26-35	36-45	46-55	56-65	65+
Excellent		49+	45+	41+	35+	31+	28+
Good	NO. OF SQUATS	40–48	36–44	31–40	26–34	22–30	20–27
Average		35-39	31–35	27–30	22–25	17–21	15–19
Fair		29–34	27–30	21–26	16–21	12–16	10–14
Poor		28-	26-	20-	15-	11-	9-

❺ Flexibility

The most commonly overlooked aspect of physical fitness is flexibility. Flexibility is the range of motion of the body's joints. Flexibility is the result of muscles, tendons, and ligaments working together. People often focus on increasing the body's muscles without taking flexibility into consideration. As muscle strength increases, the body exerts more force on the tendons and ligaments. It's important, therefore, to increase your flexibility so as to avoid injury to tendons and ligaments. You can become more flexible by stretching. Stretching should be approached with the same care and precision that you would bring to any other aspect of an exercise routine. Incorporate stretching into every workout. With increased flexibility, you will be better able to increase your strength and endurance while decreasing the chance of injury. Without proper stretching, these crucial tissues can be damaged under the new strain. Stretching enables the tendons and ligaments to handle the stress and grow with the muscles.

Sit & Reach Test: The sit and reach test measures the flexibility of your hamstrings and lower back. Before you begin, make sure you warm up. Place a ruler or tape measure on the floor with the numbers increasing away from you. Sit on the floor with your legs straight so that your heels line up with the 23-inch mark. The numbers should get higher past your heels. While seated, place your hands on top of each other and stretch forward toward your toes without bouncing. Slowly reach 3 times. On the fourth reach, record your measurement. Have someone stand over you as you reach so they can read the stretch correctly for you. The numbers listed in the table below offer median measurements. Age and arm length contribute to scoring differences.

Compare your number with the following chart.

Sit & Reach Flexibility

	SUPERIOR	EXCELLENT	GOOD	AVERAGE	POOR
MEN	27"+	25-27"	23-25"	21-23"	< 20"
WOMEN	30"+	28-30"	26-28"	24-26"	< 23"

EXERCISE & WEIGHT CONTROL

Being overweight or having too much body fat is not only a nuisance, it's bad for your health. Still, many people fight the battle of the bulge through diet alone, as exercise is not always convenient. Many people's jobs mean they spend hours behind desks and computers. In addition, much of our leisure time is spent in sedentary pursuits. To reverse this trend, it is important to adjust your attitude and find time to exercise every day.

Common excuses people use to avoid physical activity include:

1. "I don't have the time."
2. "I'm too tired and I don't feel like it."
3. "It's not convenient to get to my workout place."
4. "I'm afraid I'll look stupid and feel embarrassed."
5. "It's too expensive to join a gym."

Write down the reasons you've been avoiding exercise, joining a gym, or taking a fitness class. Now write down solutions to these reasons, which are really just excuses. For example, if your number one reason for skipping exercise is, "I don't have time," you might consider taking half your lunch break to go for a walk, or going for a bike ride with your family instead of going out to dinner.

FITNESS SOLUTIONS

EXCUSE 1:

SOLUTION 1:

EXCUSE 2:

SOLUTION 2:

EXCUSE 3:

SOLUTION 3:

There is never a good excuse to be sedentary. There are great gyms and fitness facilities of all types and price ranges. If you find the traditional gym environment isn't for you, try taking a yoga or dance class. If money is a concern, sign up for a hiking club — activities like hiking, swimming, rollerblading, and biking are always free. The website MeetUp.com is great for finding groups of people with your similar interests in your area. Flip to the next page, to the Calories Burned for Physical Activities chart, and look at how many ways there are to burn calories!

Be aware that the exact number of calories you will burn for each activity varies based on your weight. The following list is an approximation for a person weighing 150 pounds. If you weigh more, you will burn slightly more calories; if you weigh less than 150 pounds, you will burn slightly fewer calories. If you require an exact count, there are many websites that can estimate calories burned based on your weight, intensity of the workout, and the length of time you exercised.

Light Activities: 150 or Less Cal/Hr.

Billiards. 140

Lying down/sleeping 60

Office work. 140

Sitting 80

Standing 100

Moderate Activities: 150-350 Cal/Hr.

Aerobic dancing 340

Ballroom dancing 210

Bicycling (5 mph) 170

Bowling. 160

Canoeing (2.5 mph) 170

Dancing (social) 210

Gardening (moderate) 270

Golf (with cart) 180

Golf (without cart) 320

Grocery shopping 180

Horseback riding (sitting trot). 250

Light housework/cleaning, etc. 250

Pilates 240

Ping pong 270

Surfing 300

Swimming (20 yards/min). 290

Tennis (recreational doubles). 310

Vacuuming 220

Volleyball (recreational) 260

Walking (2 mph). 200

Walking (3 mph) 240

Walking (4 mph) 300

Vigorous Activities: 350 or More Cal/Hr.

Aerobics (step) 440

Backpacking (10 lb load) 540

Badminton 450

Basketball (competitive) 660

Basketball (leisure) 390

Bicycling (10 mph) 375

Bicycling (13 mph) 600

Cross country skiing (leisurely) 460

Cross country skiing (moderate) 660

Hiking 460

Ice skating (9 mph) 384

Jogging (5 mph) 550

Jogging (6 mph) 690

Racquetball 620

Rock climbing 740

Rollerblading 384

Rowing machine 540

Running (8 mph) 900

Scuba diving 570

Shoveling snow 580

Soccer 580

Spinning 650

Stair climber machine 480

Swimming (50 yards/min.) 680

Water aerobics 400

Water skiing 480

Weight training (30 sec. between sets) 760

Weight training (60 sec. between sets) 570

Yoga (Power) 400

Notes

Water & Staying Hydrated

Water is essential to survival — and to your exercise plan. Maintaining hydration is crucial for exercise weight loss. Water keeps your metabolism working hard, maintains digestion, improves muscle tone, and makes your stomach feel full. Try having a tall glass of water shortly before every meal in order to eat less.

As important as staying well hydrated is, it's easy to forget to drink water until dehydration has already set in. Research has shown that the best time to drink water is before you feel thirsty. Physical signs like dry mouth and sensations of thirst often occur only after you are already dehydrated.

How much should you drink? You need to drink at least eight 8-ounce glasses a day. That's the minimum! Men should really strive for 120 ounces of water and women should try and get 90 ounces. If you think about it, it's really not a lot. Buy a regular 750-ml aluminum water bottle (available at any store from Target to Starbucks to your local gym), fill it up 3 times, and you've already had more than 8 glasses. No matter what your ideal water consumption is, remember to increase water intake in conditions such as high heat, high altitude, low humidity, or high activity level. Water is necessary in order for metabolism to take place, so being properly hydrated helps your body turn food into the energy you need for work, family, and exercise.

Sources of Hydration

A number of liquids and solid foods can provide your body with the water it needs, including:

Water: Your body uses water most readily in its plain, unadulterated form. The bulk (80-90%) of your hydration should come from drinking plain water.

Beverages: Drinking non-caffeinated beverages, such as fruit juices, sports drinks, and milk is a good way of maintaining your hydration. Herbal teas also work well. Just remember that many beverages also contain sugar and fat, which can add unwanted calories to your diet.

Fruits and vegetables: These solid foods consist mainly of water, and therefore are excellent for hydration. Individuals who eat a healthy amount of fruits and vegetables may receive up to 20 percent of their hydration from these solid foods.

Be wary of drinking caffeinated beverages, such as coffee, tea, and many soft drinks. Caffeine is a diuretic, meaning that it stimulates your kidneys to remove water from your system. If you feel the need for a caffeinated beverage, remember to compensate by drinking extra water.

Hydration Before, During, and After Your Workout

Proper hydration is one of the easiest and most effective ways of boosting workout performance. Water is necessary for metabolism to take place, so being properly hydrated helps your body turn food into the energy you need for exercising. Water also helps your body regulate its temperature through sweating. Because vigorous exercise causes you to lose large amounts of water through sweating, it is important to drink water before, during, and after each 9-minute workout session.

Pre-workout: Drink between 8 and 16 ounces of water in the hour prior to working out.

During workout: Replenish fluids by drinking 4 to 8 ounces of water a few minutes after completing your 9-minute set.

During vigorous cardiovascular training, or if you're exercising in hot temperatures, increase your water consumption in order to replace water lost from sweating.

After workout: Drink between 8 and 16 ounces of water within 30 minutes of completing your exercise routine. Your muscles need water in order to recover from the stress of a workout. Drinking proper amounts of fluids after your workout will help reduce muscle soreness, as well as help you feel less tired.

Experts say that if your goal is to lose weight, you should increase the amount of water you consume before and after working out.

Dehydration and Performance

Just as keeping hydrated enhances physical performance, dehydration leads to decreases in physical and mental performance. When you are dehydrated, your body is unable to handle the physical exertions related to cardiovascular or strength exercises. As you become dehydrated, your blood volume can actually drop. A reduction in blood volume causes less oxygen to reach muscles, resulting in fatigue and loss of coordination. Your brain's oxygen supply is also reduced, leading to reduced concentration. Allowed to continue, dehydration can cause dizziness and even loss of consciousness.

As you work to increase your level of fitness, keep in mind that an effective workout regimen depends largely on your ability to avoid fatigue and stay focused. Keeping well hydrated will allow you to do just that.

Fitness for Health & Weight Loss

Burning Fat with Cardiovascular Exercise

Cardiovascular training focuses on improving your heart's ability to provide oxygen to your body. By requiring muscles to perform repetitious acts with only brief moments of rest, you force your heart to adapt in order to increase the amount of oxygenated blood it pumps to the muscles. This is what is known as aerobic exercise. Aerobic exercises are performed at less-than-maximum intensity in a repetitive manner for a period of time. These activities require oxygenated blood to be constantly delivered to the muscles. Through cardiovascular training, endurance increases and your body begins to maintain a higher and more efficient consumption of oxygen.

In order to improve your cardiovascular system's performance, you must determine your target heart rate, which is 50 to 85 percent of your maximum heart rate. Your target heart rate is the range at which your body is able to most efficiently burn fat and increase cardiovascular fitness.

First, to determine your maximum heart rate, enter your age into the equation below:

220 – Age = Maximum Heart Rate

For example, if you are 44 years of age, your maximum heart rate will be 176.

The following chart shows the range of target and maximum heart rates by age.

Target and Maximum Heart Rates Determined by Age

AGE	TARGET HEART RATE (50-85% OF MHR)	MAXIMUM HEART RATE
20	100-170	200
25	98-166	195
30	95-162	190
35	93-157	185
40	90-153	180
45	88-149	175
50	85-145	170
55	83-140	165
60	80-136	160
65	78-132	155
70	75-128	150

There are 3 heart rate zones that focus on specific aspects of cardiovascular performance. These 3 zones are endurance, aerobic, and anaerobic. By targeting any one of these zones, you can control the benefits you get from cardiovascular exercise. The following table illustrates the range of these zones and their benefits.

Heart Rate Zones

ZONE	% OF MAXIMUM HEART RATE	PROCESS	BENEFITS
Endurance Zone	60-70%	Burning fuel with oxygen (easy)	Builds endurance & helps with fat burning
Aerobic Zone	70-80%	Burning fuel with oxygen (intense)	Improves cardiovascular system; muscles learn to utilize oxygen more efficiently
Anaerobic Zone	80-90%	Burning fuel without oxygen	Builds heart and lung capacity

Successful Cardiovascular Training

Many find that working out in the morning gives them a boost of energy that lasts throughout the day. Others find exercising in the early evening helps prepare them for sleep. *Ultra Simple 9-Minute Workouts* gives you the benefit of both a morning and evening program. Remember, it doesn't take hours of exercise to burn fat and lose weight; it only takes consistent effort, as well as the most efficient exercises that work the heart and multiple parts of the body at once.

Footwear: Having the right shoes improves your workout and also protects you from soreness and injury. For instance, running shoes are designed for forward heel-to-toe motion, and do not provide the right ankle support for the side-to-side motion of activities like kickboxing or step aerobics. Try cross trainers, which are designed to be lightweight, and also provide traction and durability for jogging, plyometrics, weight lifting, aerobics, and more.

You may want to visit a specialty store to have your foot measured and your shoes professionally fit. A shoe should be snug but not be so tight that it puts pressure on the top of your foot or crushes your toes. And be sure to replace shoes once the soles start to get worn down or unevenly worn. Cross training shoes should be replaced once or twice a year, or every 100 hours.

Pace: The speed and intensity at which you perform the exercises in this book should be maintained at a level that does not sacrifice form or hurt any part of the body. The pace should be challenging and slightly uncomfortable, but never painful. It will be more beneficial to do fewer reps with slow, controlled movements and proper form than to perform a high number of reps with bad form, which can lead to injury.

Benefits of Strength Training

Strength training involves overloading your muscles in order to increase their strength and ability to do work. Strength training is an anaerobic activity, meaning that during this type of exercise, your muscles don't consume oxygen. These are explosive activities that focus on increasing intensity and strength. Strength training involves keeping the targeted muscles activated near or at their maximum capacity for a short period.

Strength training increases the durability of bones, muscles, tendons, and ligaments, making your body less susceptible to injury. It can also increase bone density and may help prevent osteoporosis. Recent studies have uncovered convincing evidence that strength training reduces cholesterol, resulting in a lower risk of heart disease. With the regular strength training routine in this book, you will see increases in lean muscle mass and metabolism.

In addition, stronger muscles help improve balance, mobility, and endurance. Your figure or posture will also improve as your skeletal muscles help you stand up straighter. Strength training helps bolster mental health by reducing stress and improving self-esteem. Resistance training has been proven to increase the body's production of chemicals known as neurotransmitters (dopamine, serotonin, and norepinephrine), which act in the pleasure centers of the brain, increasing feelings of contentment and well-being.

Correct Order for Training Major Muscle Groups

Ultra Simple 9-Minute Workouts includes cardio, core, upper body, and lower body programs for 3 different levels of difficulty. It is important to exercise muscles in the correct order to maximize the benefits of each exercise.

Core (abs, obliques, lower back): *Ultra Simple 9-Minute Workouts* has you performing core exercises first thing in the morning. Strong abdominal muscles will help stabilize your body so all other muscle groups can be exercised properly.

Upper Body, Back & Shoulders: You will work chest muscles, back, shoulders, triceps, and biceps in the evening. Stabilize your body with your core muscles, and perform the exercises by isolating the specific muscles being worked.

Lower Body (quadriceps, gluteus maximus, hamstring, calves): Exercising these large muscles in the evening will help promote blood flow, warming and relaxing the entire body, which is especially helpful if you sit, stand, or drive for many hours during the day.

Both the lower body and cardio programs will target the quads, glutes, hamstrings, and calves. Some will incorporate core and arm strength as well for a full-body workout.

Main Muscle Groups

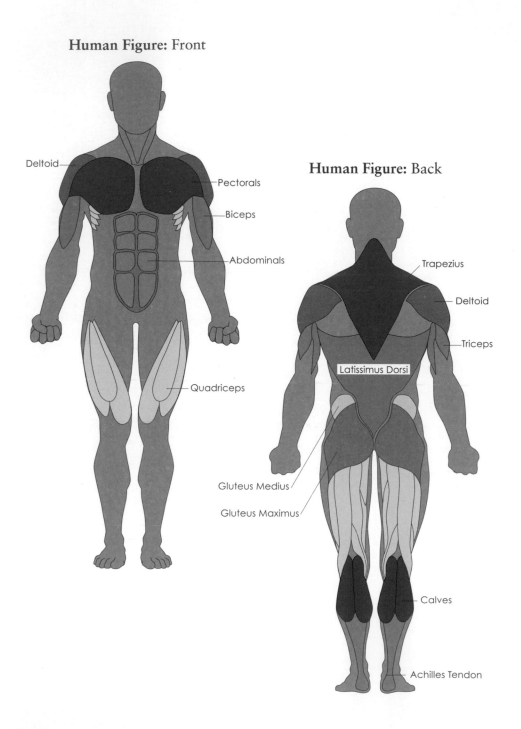

Human Figure: Front

Deltoid

Pectorals

Biceps

Abdominals

Quadriceps

Human Figure: Back

Trapezius

Deltoid

Triceps

Latissimus Dorsi

Gluteus Medius

Gluteus Maximus

Calves

Achilles Tendon

Stretching

If you're like most people, stretching is usually an after thought, an activity reserved for the "if I get around to it" part of your workout. Well, you're missing out! More and more research has proven the importance of a good hamstring stretch or neck roll for your long-term health. So what exactly is stretching doing for you? On a basic level, it's a mini workout for your muscles, making them tense up and relax, all the while forcing your veins to constrict, your blood to circulate quicker, and your heart to pump harder. Through the instant circulation boost, this seemingly futile activity actually flushes the toxins and waste out of your body, and allows more oxygen to flow to your brain (always a perk!). Also, your muscles' primary job is to constantly contract, and they achieve this function best with greater strength and length. By stretching, you are actually tearing the tiny fibers in your muscles, ligaments, and tendons. After a brief rest, your body works to repair these tears, creating stronger, longer, and more resilient body parts that are much less prone to injury. Plus, if your muscles or joints do ever become damaged, their rejuvenated selves will recover faster. Talk about a miracle fitness activity. By adding a simple stretching routine to your workout regiment, you'll begin to notice a difference in your general well-being.

Benefits of stretching

Many studies have demonstrated a direct link between stretching and a decreased risk of fitness-based injury. Think of your stretches as little personal trainers preparing your muscles and joints for future activity. As you focus on your muscles, you allow your body to practice its exercises, building the strength and range of motion it needs to, say, jog a mile, dunk a basketball, or practice a Zumba move. A regular stretching regiment will also improve your overall coordination, balance, and, of course, flexibility.

And who knew that stretching could help your mental health as well? Research connects stretching with major stress reduction. When you perform stretching exercises, your body stimulates receptors in the central nervous system that actually decrease the production of stress hormones. In addition, most people reproduce their emotional tension physically by tightening their muscles, usually in their neck and shoulders. This can spark a dull, irritating pain in your body that you might not even notice anymore. Stretching allows you to become more aware of your body's tenseness and properly release it. By engaging simple stretches a few times a day, you will relieve your mental and physical stress by making your muscles feel better, and in turn, making yourself feel better overall. So after a particularly tough day at work or a strenuous workout, ease into this rejuvenating lineup of stretches to combat your blues!

When to stretch

Pre-workout stretches can be very beneficial for enhancing your body's circulation, range of motion, coordination, and flexibility. However, it is important to engage in a warm up before you head to the mats. Never start stretching "cold" muscles, or you will increase the risk of pulling a muscle or making previous injuries worse. Simple warm ups include jumping jacks, a quick jaunt on the treadmill, or low-intensity biking for 5-10 minutes.

Many fitness trainers also encourage stretching directly following your workout, when you know your muscles have truly warmed up. Stretching after high levels of activity ensures you are lengthening and building resilience in those recently used muscles, balancing out the recent strain you just placed on them.

Before and after your workout, you should try 3 to 5 of the stretches highlighted below this section. Hold them for 10 to 20 seconds each. To make the most out of your stretching time, be sure to alternate your stretches, and try to use examples that relate to the area you plan to or have already addressed during your workout.

Stretching Dos and Don'ts:

Do:
- Remember to breathe slowly and evenly while you stretch.
- Make sure your muscles are warm before you stretch them by engaging in a quick warm up.
- Relax while you stretch, as it will improve your flexibility and ease tension.
- Avoid pain! Stretching should not hurt.
- Be sure to hold your stretch for at least 10 seconds.
- Stretch in a circular fashion to increase the range of motion in your joints.

Don't:
- Make sure not to hold your breathe, as this will only cause injury and unnecessary tension.
- Don't favor any particular side or muscle group when you stretch. Ensure each side gets the same amount of time.
- Make sure not to bounce or rock while you are stretching. Slow, easy movement is the key to improving your flexibility.
- Don't overstretch by pulling or pushing harder then your muscles allow in any particular direction.

Waist and Lower Spine

Lie on the floor with your arms out to the side. Bring your left hand down and your right knee up. Place your left hand on your knee and turn your hips to the left. Use your hand to help push your knee down as close to the ground as is comfortable. Keep your right hand extended and your left leg straight.

Hold this stretch for 10 seconds while gently pressing your knee to the floor, easing up as needed. Switch sides and repeat.

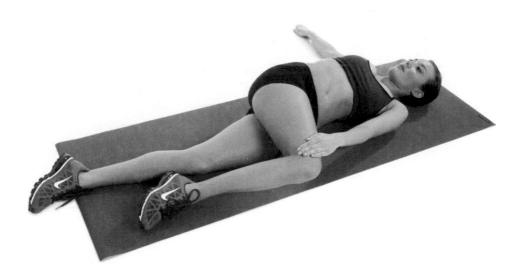

Side Bend

Stand tall. Reach one hand above your head and reach to the other side of the room over the ear. Hold for 10 to 15 seconds. You should feel a stretch up the side of the body. Switch sides and repeat.

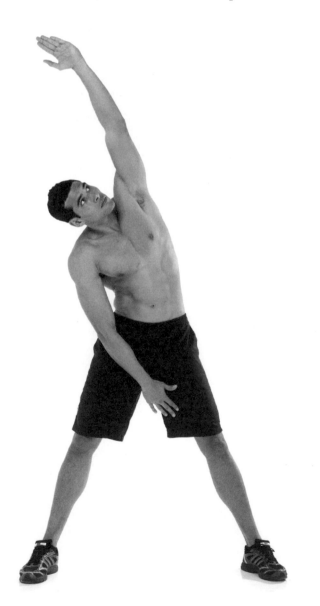

Tricep Stretch

Put one arm overhead and bend so the palm is reaching down the upper back. Grasp elbow overhead with other hand and pull elbow back and down. Hold for 10 to 15 seconds. You should feel a stretch in the back of the upper arm. Repeat with opposite arm.

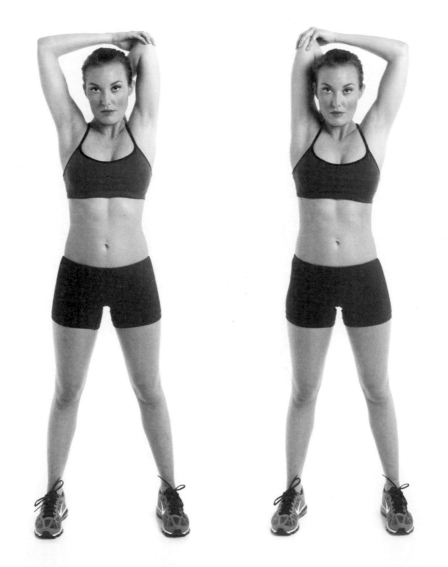

Deltoid Stretch

Reach one arm across your chest, and hold it in place with the other arm. Hold for 10 to 15 seconds. You should feel a stretch in your upper back muscle. Stretch each arm.

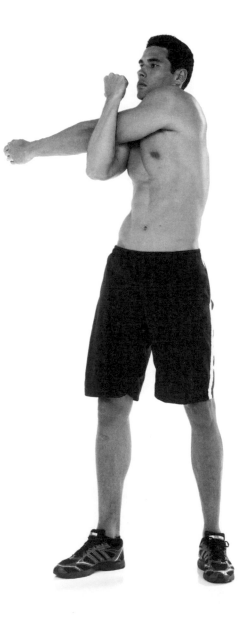

Inner Thigh Stretch (Butterfly)

Begin seated on the floor. Bend your legs and let the knees drop to the side with the soles of your feet touching, in a butterfly position.

Pull your heels toward you while pushing your knees toward the floor. Hold for 30 seconds.

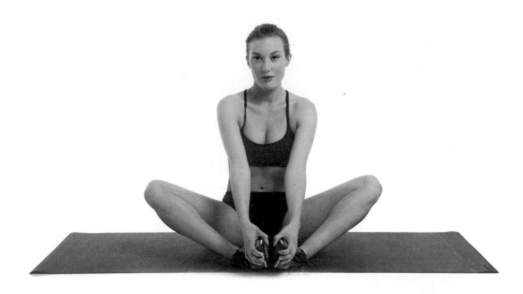

Neck Rolls

Stand with feet shoulder-width apart. Roll your neck in a circular motion in one direction about 10 times. Switch, and roll in the opposite direction 10 times.

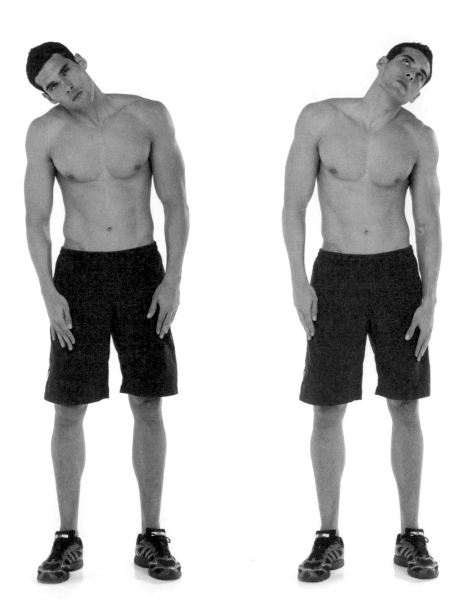

Calf Stretch

Start on the floor with your hands below your shoulders and your knees below your hips. Next, straighten your legs and push off the floor, raising your hips and bottom in the air.

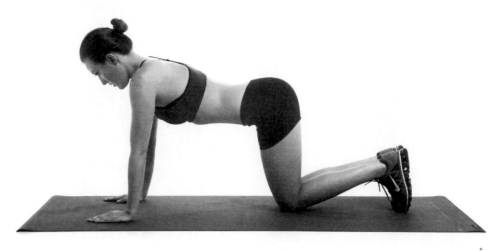

Keep your legs straight and gently try and ease your heels to the floor. Hold for 10 seconds and return to start position for a rest.

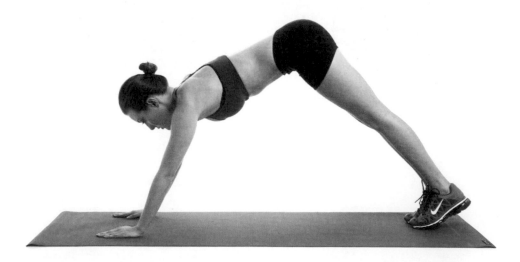

Glute Stretch

Stand tall, pulling the knee up to the chest and holding it there. You should feel the stretch in the back of your thigh and glute. Stretch both legs for the same amount of time.

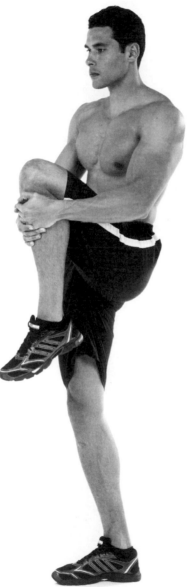

Sitting Hamstring Stretch

Sit on the floor with your back straight and arms at rest in front of you. Slowly, lean forward while keeping your back straight. Raise your arms and try to touch your toes.

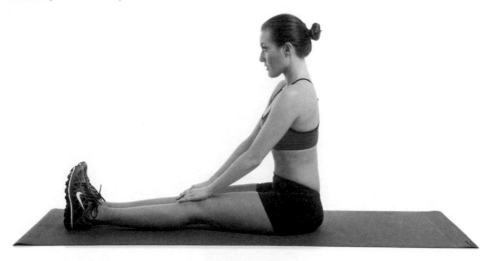

Ease forward as far as you can go and hold for 10 seconds. Then return to starting position.

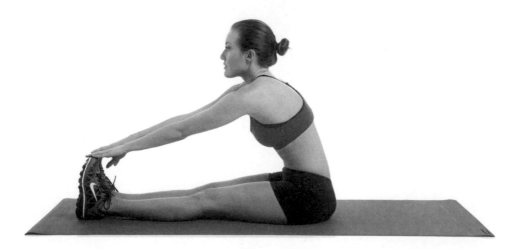

Quad Stretch

Stand tall, pulling one heel up to the glute, and holding the foot with your hand. Hold the stretch, feeling it in the front of the thigh. Stretch both legs.

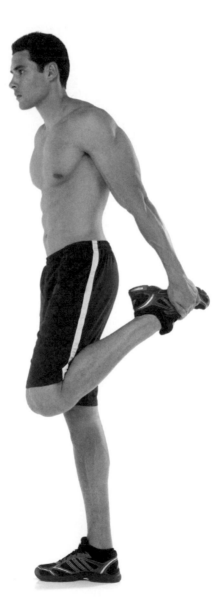

Notes

Ultra Simple 9-Minute Workouts

Ultra Simple 9-Minute Workout Plan

Losing weight requires a fitness plan full of high-intensity, calorie-blasting exercises that work the entire body. The *Ultra Simple 9-Minute Workouts* exercise plan is designed to target multiple muscle groups, build core strength, and get the heart rate elevated to burn body fat.

For 6 days each week, you will pair a strength training circuit with cardio or core exercises. You will switch off every day between a lower body and core strength training circuit, and an upper body and cardio strength training circuit. Give your body a rest on the last day of the week — you deserve it!

Every strength training exercise comes with step-by-step instructions so you can ensure you are performing every activity with the correct form, without risking injury.

The Benefits of this Program

The beauty of the *Ultra Simple 9-Minute Workouts* exercise plan is, as the name suggests, it only takes 9 minutes out of your mornings and evenings. And, the activities are designed to be performed anywhere, including in the comfort of your own living room (yes that's right — you now have that "home gym" you always wanted). Long gone are the days of skipping a fitness routine simply because you don't have time to hit the local gym or step out for a long run. Now you can exercise while your morning coffee brews. De-stress after a long day at work by engaging in the evening routine while watching your favorite sitcom. You could even make it a family activity and include the kids. You'll be surprised to find how just 18 minutes a day makes a huge impact on your health and appearance.

Variety is the Spice of Life

The same routine for anything gets stale after awhile. As *Ultra Simple 9-Minute Workouts* program schedule makes you vary the types of exercises and targeted muscle groups every time, you reduce the possibility of boredom and plateauing. By combining cardio with strength training and core exercises, you'll hit every key body area, while looking forward to trying out the next new moves in your schedule.

How to Perform the Exercise Plan

6 days a week, set aside about 9 minutes to complete this workout plan in the mornings and evenings. Perform each exercise for 50 seconds, with as many reps as you can do in that time without sacrificing form. Take a 10-second rest to get ready for the next exercise. Keep an eye on a stopwatch, timer on an mp3 player, or clock with a seconds hand. Complete all 3 exercises in the circuit. Do the same for the evening circuit. The last day of each week is reserved for rest and relaxation (and congratulating yourself on a week well spent, of course!).

Warming Up and Cooling Down

Always begin and end your workouts with a 5 to 10-minute warm up and cool down. Warm ups and cool downs are vital steps to any fitness routine, as they prevent tear and strain, as well as adhere to your heart's well-being. Walk to loosen the muscles. Next, stretch to prepare your muscles for work and prevent injury. Be sure to take advantage of the important stretches shown in the previous chapter. The same routine after your workout will bring the heart rate down, help the body recover, and prevent soreness.

Your Workout Schedule

You have 9 weeks to get the body you've always wanted, so work hard and push yourself, even if it's to do just 1 more rep each time! You'll love the success and pride you'll feel after a tough workout. The body, strength, and shape you've always wanted are just weeks away.

DAY	MORNING	EVENING
Mon	Core	Lower Body
Tues	Cardio	Upper Body
Wed	Core	Lower Body
Thurs	Cardio	Upper Body
Fri	Core	Lower Body
Sat	Cardio	Upper Body
Sun	Rest Day!	Rest Day!

Notes

Ultra Simple 9-Minute Workouts

Core Exercises

Equipment:

Stability ball
Dumbbell

Strength training is a very important part of losing weight. The following workout will lengthen and tone your core while replacing body fat with muscle (which burns 3 times as many calories as fat!).

The exercises in this section work all parts of the core, including the abs, obliques, and lower back. You'll also work the arms, shoulders, and more. When coupled with a cardio program, these moves will help you get in shape quickly. Plus, they're fun and challenging!

Crunch On A Stability Ball

level 1

 Start with your shoulders, lower back, and hips on a stability ball. Interlace your fingers behind your head, and pull your belly button in toward your spine.

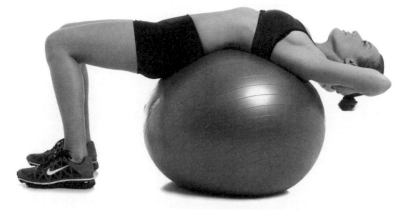

 Raise your head and shoulders in a crunch, pausing at the top, and returning slowly to the start position.

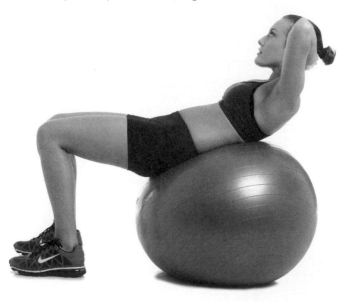

Plank with Reach

level 1

 Get into plank position, with elbows directly under shoulders, and feet spread slightly wider than your hips.

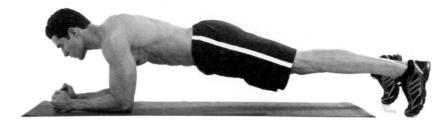

 Keeping your core engaged, reach forward and out with your right arm. Hold for a second, and then return to starting position. Switch arms.

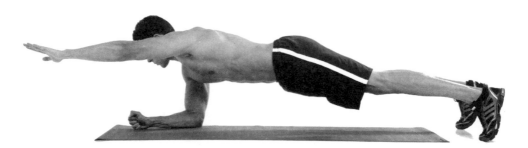

Hip Crossover with stability ball

level 1

1 Rest your feet on a stability ball with knees bent, so the ball is resting against the back of the thighs. Arms should be straight out to the sides.

2 Squeezing the ball against the backs of the thighs and engaging the core, drop the ball to the right side, as low as you can without lifting your shoulders off the floor.

3 Reverse the movement all the way to the left side, without pausing in the middle, to complete 1 rep. Then return to center and repeat.

Bird Dog

level 1

 Start in a table position, with your hands and knees on the floor shoulder-width apart. Keep your core engaged so the hips don't sag, and the back doesn't arch.

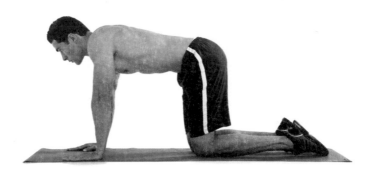

 Raise your right arm out in front and your left leg back simultaneously, keeping them in line with your torso. Hold for a second, then return to the starting position. Repeat with the opposite arm and leg.

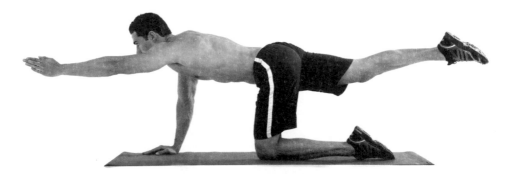

Side Bend with Dumbbell

level 1

 1 Stand straight with your feet shoulder-width apart, holding a dumbbell in each hand, palms facing your sides.

 2 Keeping your back straight and bending only at the waist, bend to one side as far as you can, feeling your oblique muscles engage on both sides. Then return to the starting position and repeat. Repeat on the same side, switching at the 25-second mark.

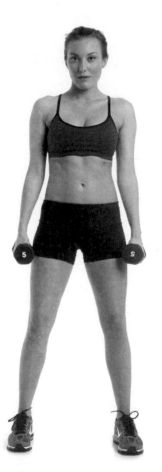

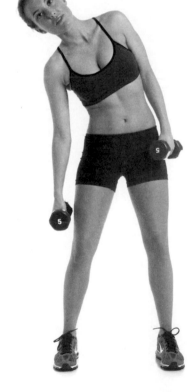

Beetle Crunch

level 1

 Lie on your back, raise your knees, and interlace your hands behind your head (as you would for a traditional crunch). Draw your belly button toward your spine and crunch off the floor and to your right, reaching your right elbow to your right thigh.

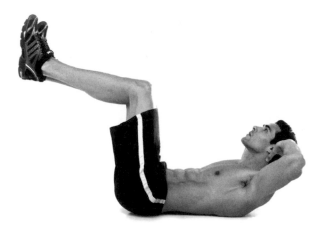

 Pause in the crunch, and then lower back down, keeping your shoulders lifted off the floor the entire time. Repeat, alternating sides.

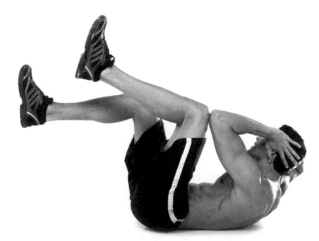

X Sit-ups

level 2

 Lie on your back with arms and legs stretched out slightly wider than shoulder-width apart, forming am X-shape. Then fold your left hand behind your head.

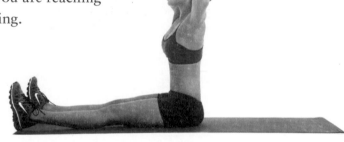

 Sit straight up, pointing your right hand up above the head as if you are reaching for the ceiling.

 Next, crunch forward, reaching the right hand across the body to touch the left toe. Reverse the movement and lie back down for 1 rep. Switch arms and repeat on the opposite side.

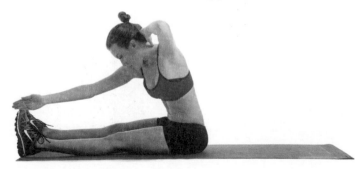

Bicycles

level 2

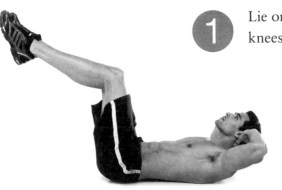

1 Lie on your back with your knees bent at a 90-degree angle.

2 Lace your fingers behind your head. Lift your head and shoulders, exhale, and twist to one side, bringing your knee in to touch your opposite elbow, while straightening the other leg. Return to center, inhale.

3 Exhale and twist to the opposite side.

Reverse Crunch

level 2

 Lie on your back with your arms by your sides. Keep your palms pressed into the floor and bend your knees at a 90-degree angle.

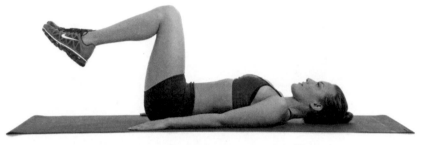

 Lift your pelvis, using the lower abs, and hollow out the belly. Your knees should come slightly in toward your head. Pause at the top of the crunch, then lower the legs just above the floor for 1 rep.

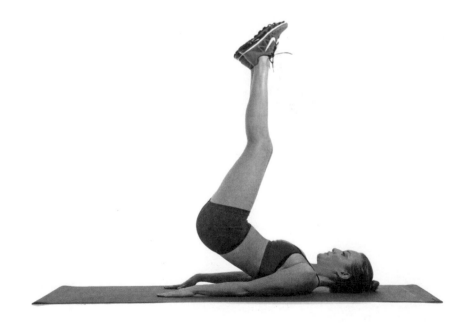

Toe Reach Crunch

level 2

 Lie on your back and lift your arms and legs straight up in the air.

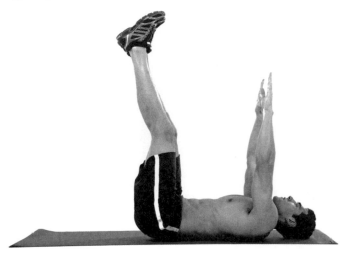

 Crunch up using the lower abs, as if you were reaching for your toes. Your head, neck, and shoulders should come off the ground. Lower for 1 rep.

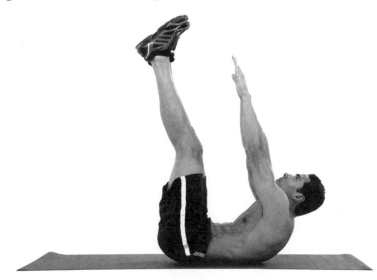

Side Plank w/ Hip Raise

level 2

 Prop yourself up into a plank position, with knees straight out, hips lifted, and your elbow and forearm on the floor directly under the shoulder. Feet should be stacked one on top of the other. Your body should form a straight line.

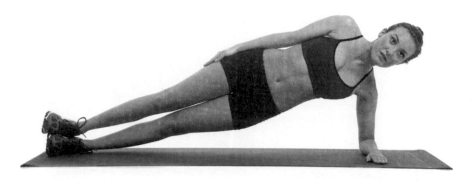

 Engaging the core, lower the hips toward the floor, pause, and lift them back so your body is straight again for 1 rep. Continue to lower and raise the hips. Switch sides at the 25-second mark.

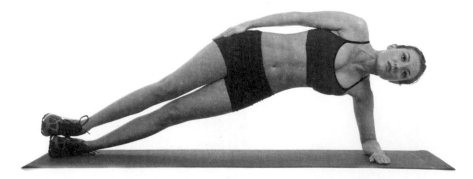

Side Crunch

level 2

 Lie on your back and interlace your fingers behind your head. Bend your knees at a 90-degree angle, and drop them to one side without twisting your upper body.

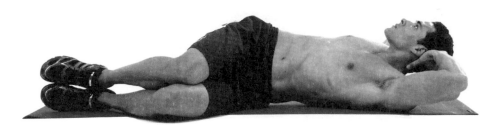

 Lift your shoulder off the floor, crunching toward your feet. Pause at the top of the crunch, then lower for 1 rep.

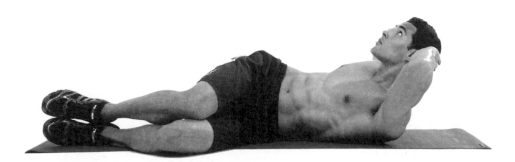

Rollout On A Stability Ball

level 3

 Kneel in front of a stability ball. Interlace your fingers tightly and place your fist on the top of the ball.

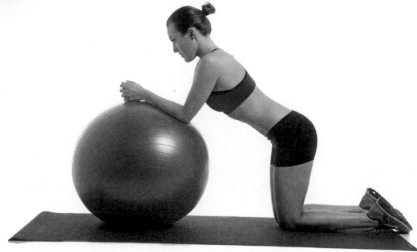

 Keeping your core engaged, slowly roll the ball out and away from you, straightening your arms as much as you can without sagging your hips or collapsing through the lower back. Use your abs to pull yourself back to the starting position.

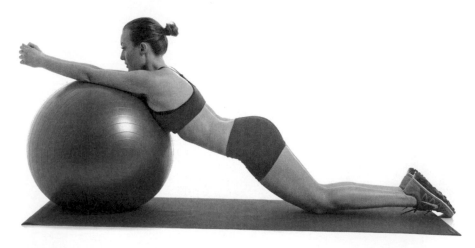

V-Up

level 3

 Lie on the floor with arms stretched above the head, and legs straight out in front.

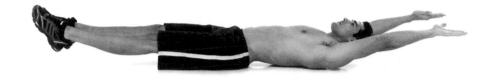

 Simultaneously lift your chest and legs straight up, reaching the fingers toward the toes. Lower back to the ground for 1 rep.

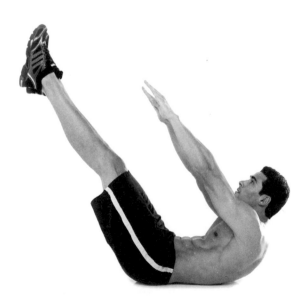

Jackknife Pike on Ball

level 3

 Begin in a plank position with your hands under your shoulders, and the tops of the feet and shins elevated on a stability ball.

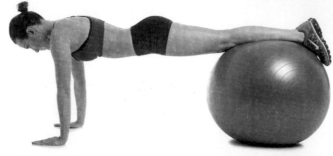

 Without rounding the lower back, lift your hips so you end up in a pike position with straight legs. Using your core muscles, pull the ball in toward the body.

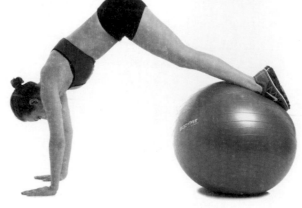

 Push the ball back out to plank to complete 1 rep.

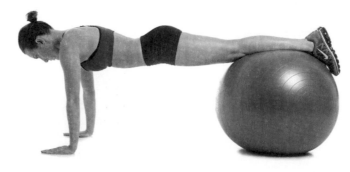

Superman Roll

level 3

1 Lie flat on your stomach with your arms straight out in front of you and legs straight out behind you, both about shoulder-width apart. Lift your legs and arms simultaneously at least 6 inches off the ground.

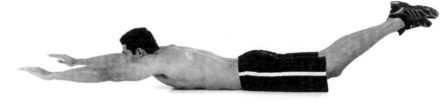

2 In a fluid motion, roll onto your back, keeping your arms and legs elevated off the ground, and engaging the core. Reach your arms and legs away from the body, lengthening the core.

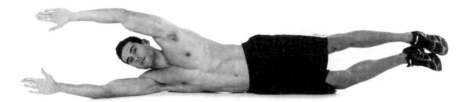

3 Continue to roll back and forth, pausing after each roll, until you need to rest.

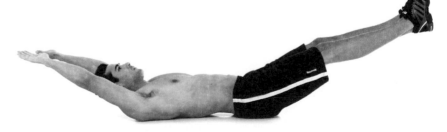

Side Plank With Push-up

level 3

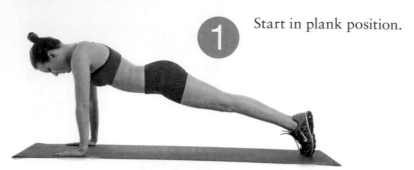

1 Start in plank position.

2 Flip to one side; straighten your bottom arm directly under your shoulder, legs straight, and feet stacked. Place your free hand on your hip or stretch it upwards. Keep your back straight and do not allow your hips to sag. Work on tightening your abs and lifting your side away from the ground.

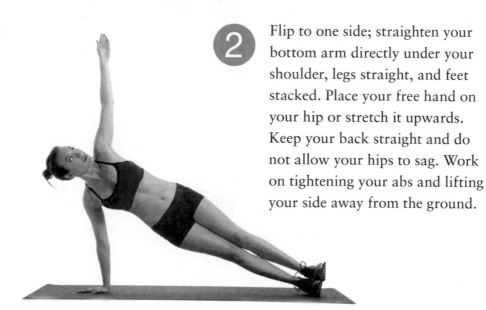

3 Flip back to plank and complete a push-up for 1 rep on that side. Repeat, switching sides.

Russian Twist With A Dumbbell

level 3

1 Sit upright with your legs bent and feet lifted off the floor. Hold a dumbbell with both hands against your chest. Lean slightly back so your upper body forms a 45-degree angle with the floor.

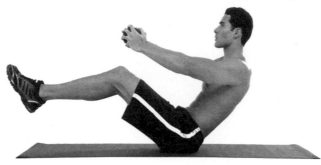

2 Rotate your arms and the dumbbell as far to one side as you can, reaching down while you squeeze your abs and obliques.

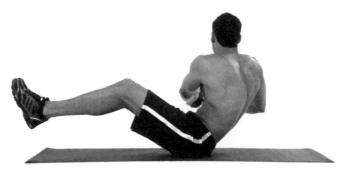

3 Return to center and twist to the other side. Rotate from your core, not your hips.

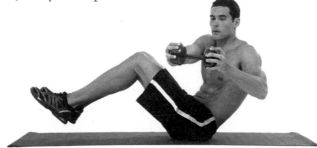

Notes

Ultra Simple 9-Minute Workouts

Lower Body

This series of lunges, raises, and plyometric moves will whip your thighs, hamstrings, glutes, and calves into shape in no time! You'll feel stronger and more explosive throughout the entire lower body.

A lower body circuit combined with cardio work can be a lot on the legs, so be sure to walk for a few minutes or jog in place to warm up the body completely. And remember, concentrate on using proper form to make the most of these moves.

Side Leg Raise

level 1

 Lie down on your left side and rest your head in the crook of your elbow. Place your right hand in front of your body for stability.

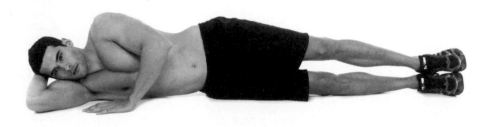

 Keeping your body still, use the inner and outer thigh muscles, as well as the glutes to lift your right leg straight up as high as you can. Pause for a second at the top, then lower the leg to the starting position. Repeat, switching legs at the 25-second mark.

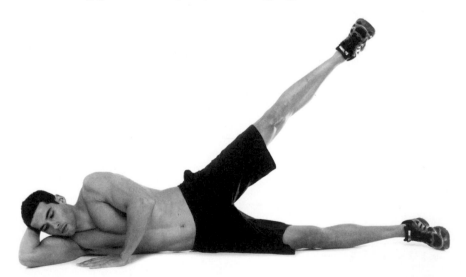

Fire Hydrant

level 1

1 Get on your hands and knees with a flat back, in a table position.

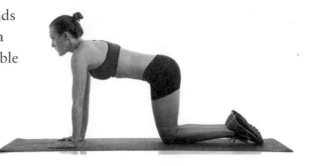

2 Keeping your knee bent, lift one knee up and out to the side. Try to lift the knee as high as your hip, or whatever height is comfortable, squeezing the glutes.

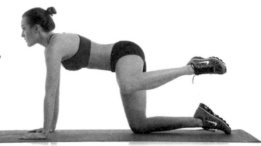

3 Next, kick the raised leg back until it is straight behind you. Lower the leg to the starting position. Repeat, switching legs at the 25-second mark.

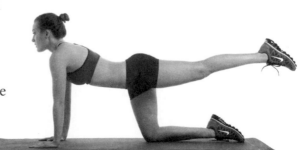

Body Weight Squat

level 1

1 Stand tall with your feet shoulder-width apart. Engage your core and lift your arms straight out in front of your chest.

2 Keeping your torso as upright as possible, bend your knees and push your hips back as you lower into a squat. Keep your weight in your heels, and aim to get the tops of your thighs parallel to the ground. Pause for a second in the squat, then push back up through your heels to return to a standing position.

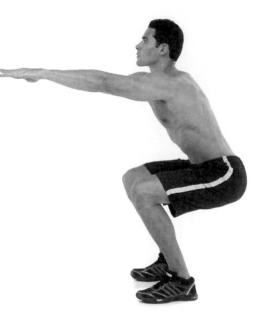

Bridge Pose

level 1

 Lie flat with knees bent hip-width apart; tuck your pelvis so your lower back touches the floor. Place your feet as close to your body as you can comfortably.

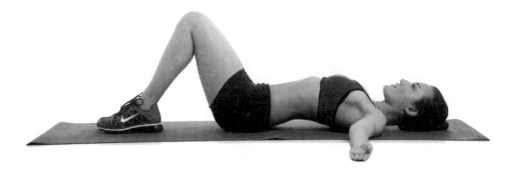

 Raise your hips until your body forms a straight line from shoulders to knees. Squeeze your glutes and lift through the thighs. Hold for 2 seconds and lower to the floor for 1 rep.

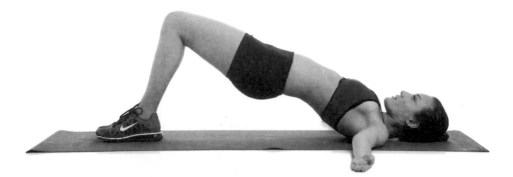

Genie Sits

level 1

 Kneel on a mat with feet together, knees slightly apart. Fold your arms over your chest.

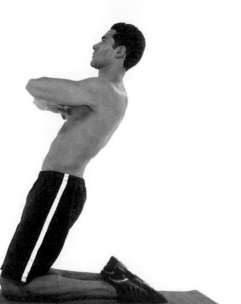

 Keeping the core engaged and back straight, lean backward as far as you can without feeling a pinch in the lower back.

 Pause; then use the front of your thighs and your core to pull you forward to the starting position.

Walking Lunges

level 1

1 Stand upright, feet together, with your hands on your hips. Take a step forward with your left leg and lunge so your hips lower toward the floor. Your front knee should come to a 90-degree angle (the knee should not go past the foot).

2 Push through the back foot and step forward to the starting position for 1 rep. Now, walk another step forward and repeat with the right leg at the front of the lunge. Travel forward until you run out of space, and then come back in the opposite direction.

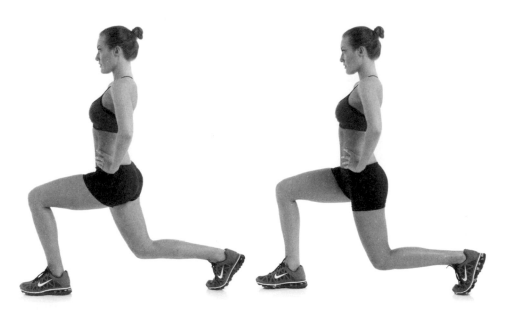

Lunges With A Twist

level 2

 Start standing, holding a dumbbell in both hands. Step forward into a lunge, making sure your knee doesn't go past your toes.

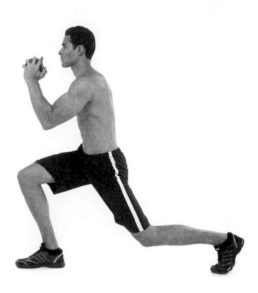

 When you reach the lowest point of your lunge, twist your torso to the side of the leg that is up, squeezing the core. Stand up from the lunge and repeat on the other leg.

Twisting Arabesque

level 2

1 In your right hand, hold a light dumbbell on one end. Stand with your arms at your sides. Place your right toe on the floor about a foot behind you.

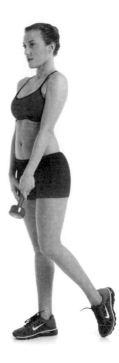

2 Bend forward from the hips. Keeping your right leg straight, raise it off the floor until your body forms a T, and your arms hang straight down from your shoulders. Your left knee can have a slight bend for stability.

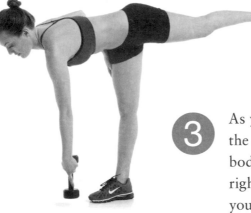

3 As you bend forward, twist from the core and reach across the body, so the dumbbell in your right hand comes down toward your left foot. Return to the starting position. Switch legs and hold the dumbbell in the other hand at the 25-second mark.

Plié Squat w/ Pulse

level 2

 Stand with your feet slightly wider than shoulder-width apart and toes turned out. Keeping your torso as upright as possible, lower your body toward the floor in a plié squat. Sink as low as you can without letting your knees go past your toes. Be sure to tuck your tailbone under so your butt doesn't stick out.

 At the lowest point in your plié squat, pulse up and down twice, contracting your inner thighs and glutes. Then, lift back up to a standing position, pushing through your heels and inner thighs, to complete 1 rep.

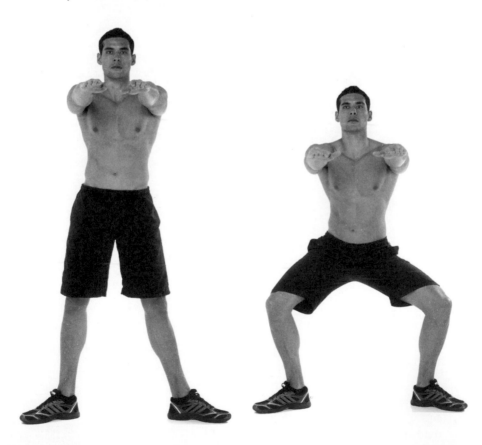

One Leg Hip Raise

level 2

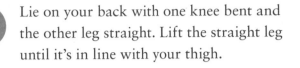

1 Lie on your back with one knee bent and the other leg straight. Lift the straight leg until it's in line with your thigh.

2 Lift your hips upward, keeping your left leg elevated. Pause; then slowly lower your hips and leg back to the starting position on the ground. Switch legs at the 25-second mark.

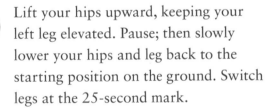

Side Lunge With Chop

level 2

1 Stand with legs shoulder-width apart and toes slightly turned out, holding a dumbbell on both ends at chest-height.

2 Lunge to the right side, bringing the dumbbell across the front of the body and down toward the outer edge of the foot.

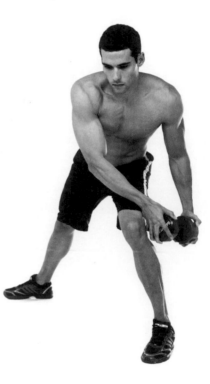

3 Press back up through the foot and thigh to return to a standing position. Repeat until the 25-second mark. Switch sides.

Clamshell w/ Dumbbell

level 2

 Lie on your side with your knees slightly bent and legs and heels together. Rest your head against the crook of your elbow. Rest your top arm against your hip and leg, holding a dumbbell comfortably against the hip area to create resistance and added difficulty.

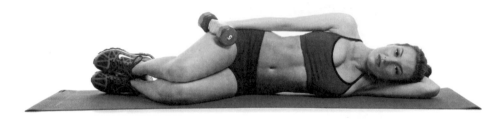

 Keeping your feet and heels together, raise your top knee as high as you can, mimicking the shape of a clamshell. Pause at the top of the movement, then lower to start position. Switch sides at the 25-second mark.

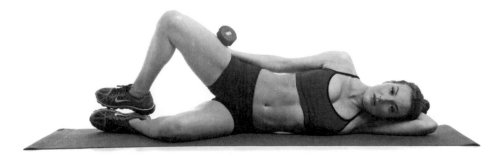

Squat & Kick

level 3

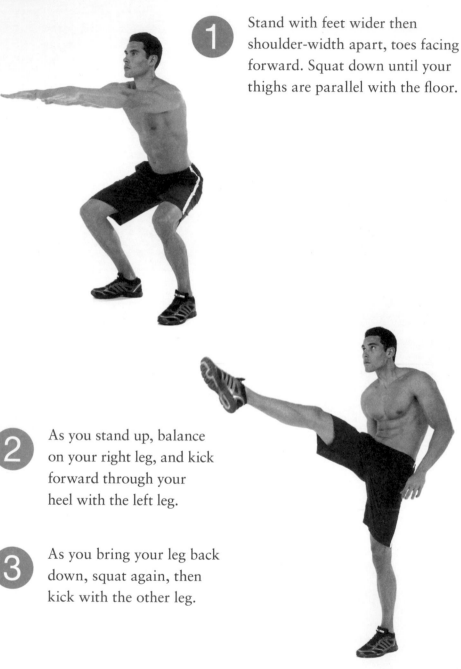

1 Stand with feet wider then shoulder-width apart, toes facing forward. Squat down until your thighs are parallel with the floor.

2 As you stand up, balance on your right leg, and kick forward through your heel with the left leg.

3 As you bring your leg back down, squat again, then kick with the other leg.

Sumo Squats With Dumbbell

level 3

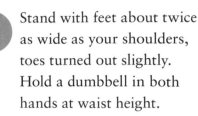

1 Stand with feet about twice as wide as your shoulders, toes turned out slightly. Hold a dumbbell in both hands at waist height.

2 Squat as low as you can, keeping a natural arch in the lower back as if you are going to touch the weight to the ground between your feet.

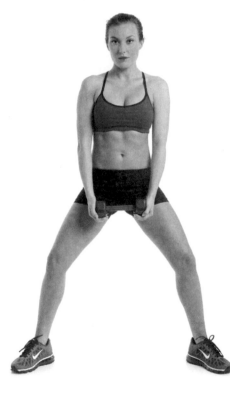

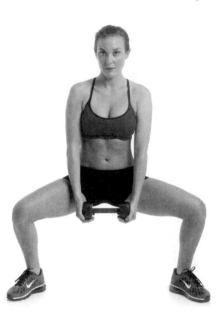

3 Come back up to the starting position and repeat. Keep the core engaged, focus the weight into your heels, and squeeze your glutes as you rise, pushing with the toes to work the calves as well.

Single Leg Dip

level 3

 Stand on your left foot. Bend your right knee and lift your right foot behind you so the lower leg is parallel to the floor.

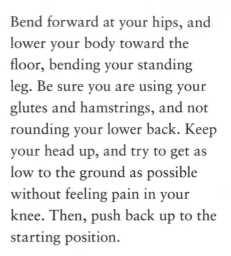 Bend forward at your hips, and lower your body toward the floor, bending your standing leg. Be sure you are using your glutes and hamstrings, and not rounding your lower back. Keep your head up, and try to get as low to the ground as possible without feeling pain in your knee. Then, push back up to the starting position.

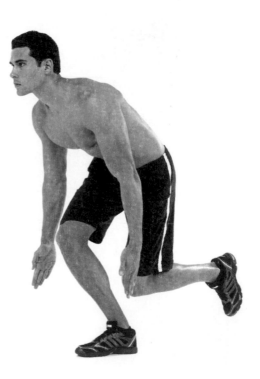

Bridge Pose And Curl On Stability Ball

level 3

1 Lie on your back with your feet and calves resting on a stability ball. Have your arms resting easily out to the sides.

2 Using your core and glutes, lift your hips off the ground so your body forms a straight line.

3 Curl the stability ball in toward your butt with your heels, as close as you can get it without arching your lower back. Your hips should stay in line with your body. Then, slide the ball back out, and lower the hips to the ground for 1 rep.

Crossover Lunge & Overhead Press

level 3

 Stand with your feet hip-width apart. Hold 2 dumbbells with your arms straight down, palms facing toward your sides.

 Keeping your back upright and hips and shoulders square, take a big step back with your right leg, crossing it behind your left. Bend your knees and lower your hips until your left thigh is nearly parallel to the floor.

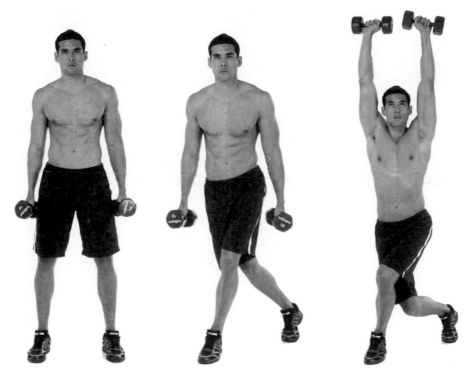

 At the bottom of the lunge, press the dumbbells up overhead to touch end to end, palms facing outward. Lower the dumbbells and step up from the lunge to return to the starting position.

Farmer's Walk on Toes

level 3

 1 Grab the heaviest pair of weights you can hold comfortably, with your arms down by your sides.

 2 Standing as tall as you can with your chest out, rise up onto the toes and the balls of the feet. Walk in a circle or a line for the full 50 seconds, keeping your heels up the entire time.

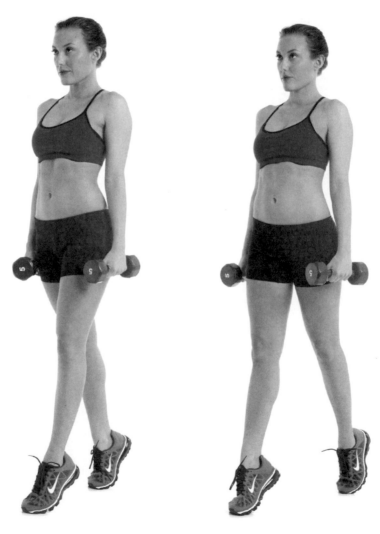

Notes

Cardio

Equipment:

Stability ball
Dumbbell

Combining strength training with cardiovascular exercise is the best way to lose weight quickly, safely, and easily. Cardio is considered the superstar of your fitness routine, burning calories, increasing your lung capacity, reducing stress and depression, as well as building and toning muscle. The best part? Cardio keeps you healthy, combating the risk of heart attack, high cholesterol, diabetes, and even some cancers.

And contrary to popular belief, running isn't the only way to get your heart pumping. Cardio should never be boring, so use the following simple, convenient exercises to spice it up. Just remember — aim to get to your target heart rate zone, or 50 to 85 % of your maximum heart rate, in order to burn fat. You should work up a sweat but still be able to talk. Now hop to it!

Jumping Jacks

level 1

 Stand with feet together and arms by your sides.

 Jump legs out to the sides, simultaneously raising arms overhead; then immediately jump back to the starting position. Repeat as fast as you can, focusing on controlling the arms and legs.

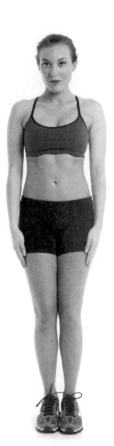

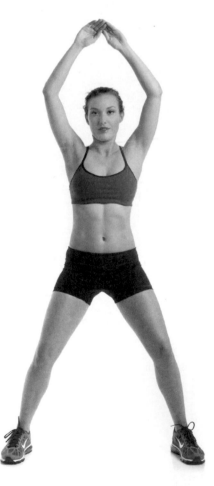

Jog in Place

level 1

 Start standing. Engage your core and start pumping your arms and legs, jogging in place to get the heart rate up.

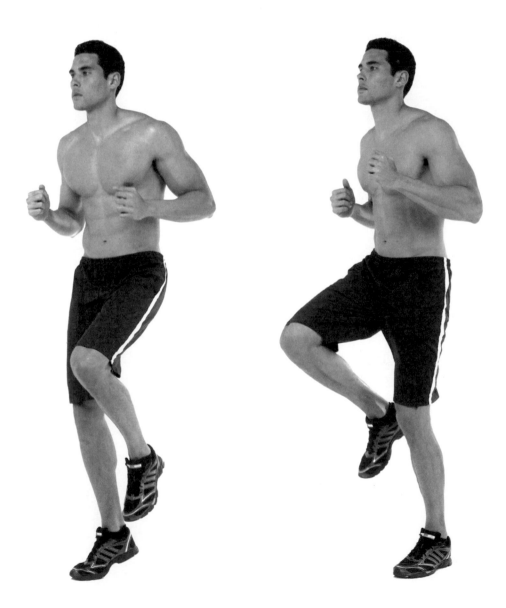

Hamstring Curl

level 1

 Start standing tall. Step sideways with right foot. Bring the left heel in toward the glute, pulling your elbows in to your sides. Reverse the motion.

 Alternate legs in a fluid motion, without pausing between sides.

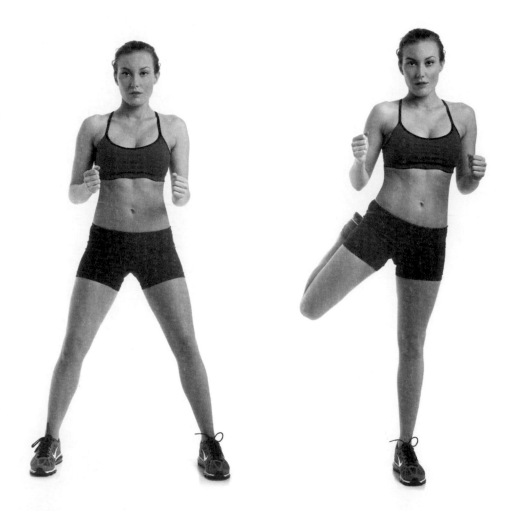

Knee Kick

level 1

 Begin in fighting stance, with the kicking leg back.

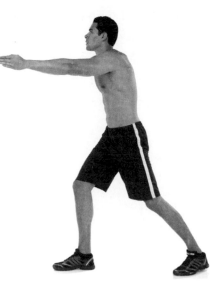

 Reaching up with your arms as if you are pulling an imaginary opponent toward you, drive your knee up, keeping your toes pointed and in line with your shin. Bend your bottom leg slightly for balance. Drop the kicking leg back down, and repeat, alternating legs.

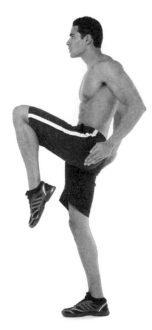

Bob and Weave

level 1

 Stand with feet wider than shoulder-width apart, knees slightly bent. Bend your arms, make fists, and bring your hands up in front of you like a boxer.

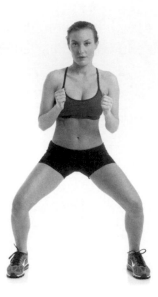

 Squat down and push off from side to side in a fluid motion, as if you were dipping under an imaginary bar. Keep the chest and head lifted, and core engaged.

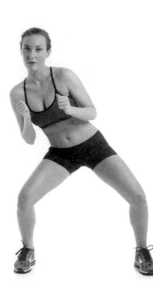

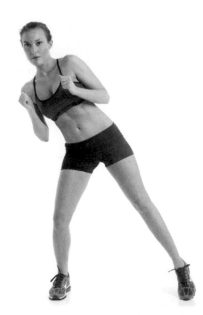

Long Jump

level 1

 Start standing, with feet together. Bend your knees into a slight squat to get power into your legs, preparing for the jump.

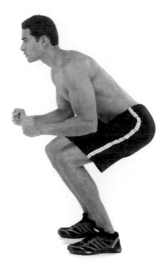

 Pumping your arms, jump forward as far as you can, landing on both feet with knees bent. Never lock your knees on the landing. Turn around and jump back the way you came.

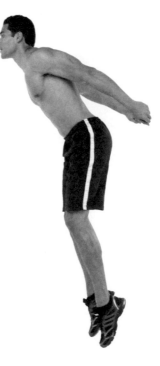

Jump Rope No Rope

level 2

 Grab your imaginary jump rope and stand tall. Begin jumping on your toes as if skipping over a rope. Rotate your arms as if holding a jump rope. Keep your core engaged and generate power through the calves, thighs, and glutes.

 At the 25-second mark, switch to alternating legs, keeping your knees down and feet kicking back toward the glutes.

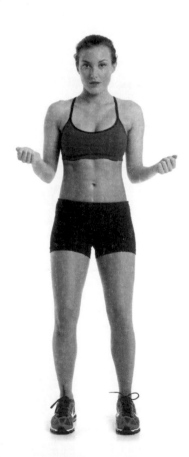

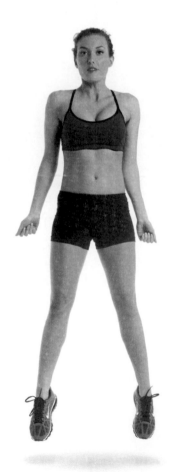

Uppercut

level 2

 1 Start in fighting stance, holding your arms with elbows bent and close to your body.

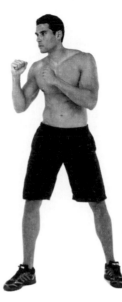

 2 Get low for power and step into the punch, pushing your left fist up. Remember to push through your legs and core.

3 Recoil and repeat, switching arms halfway through at the 25-second mark.

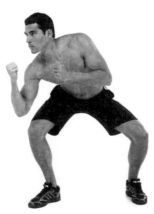

Star Jumps

level 2

 Stand with your knees slightly bent.

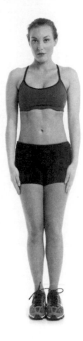

 Squat down and get ready to explode up and out.

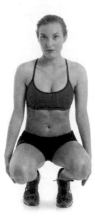

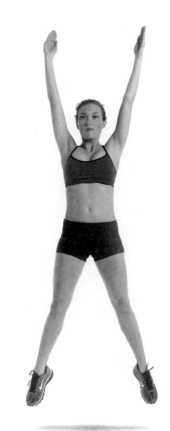

 Jump as high as you can, stretching your arms and legs out to the sides in a star shape. Before you land, pull your arms and legs back in to your body, returning to the starting position. Repeat with little to no rest between jumps.

Front Kick

level 2

 Start with left foot forward in a fighting stance, fists up. Begin to shift your weight to the left foot.

2 Kick straight out as if you were reaching with the ball of the foot. Retract immediately and return to fighting stance. Switch to the other leg halfway through at the 25-second mark.

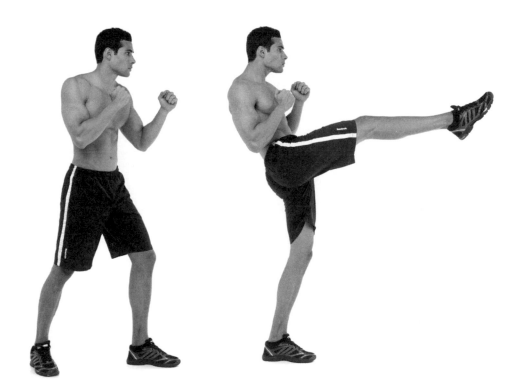

High Knees

level 2

 Bend your arms at 90-degree angles and hold them out in front of you, palms down.

 Start running in place on your toes, lifting the knees as high as your palms. Make sure you don't lean back or round your back. Repeat as fast as you can.

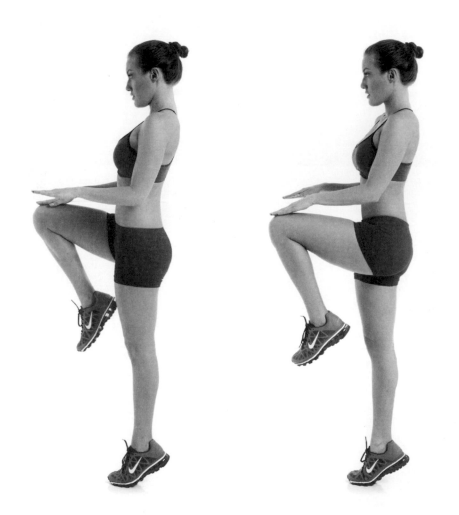

Four Corners Jump

level 2

 Stand with knees slightly bent and visualize a square shape on the floor where you will be jumping to each corner. First, jump forward about 2 feet.

 Next, jump to the right side the same distance.

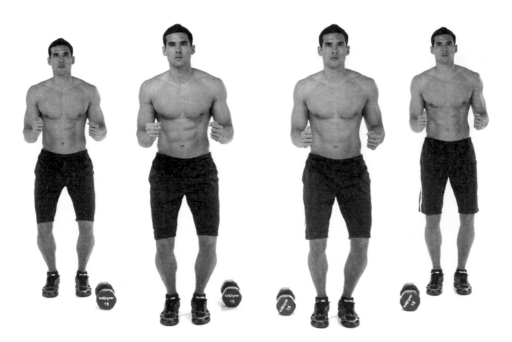

 Now, jump backward about 2 feet.

4 Finally, jump to the left side, landing back approximately in the spot where you started, completing the full square. Perform the next rep in the opposite direction, jumping right, front, left, and back. Alternate direction each time.

Split Jumps

level 3

 Start in a low lunge stance.

 Bend the knees and jump up, switching legs to land in the same position on the opposite leg. Go as quickly as you can without sacrificing form.

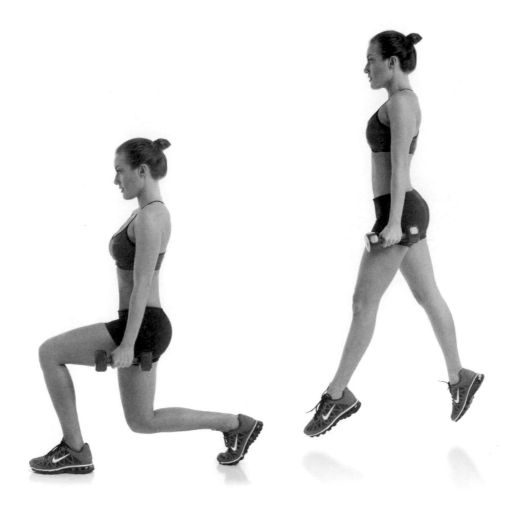

Mountain Climbers

level 3

 Begin in a push-up position with arms straight. Bring one knee in towards the chest, placing the toes on the floor.

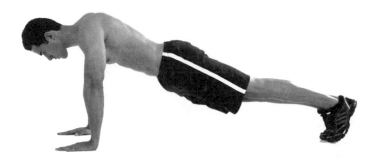

 Jump and switch legs in the air, bringing the back foot forward and the front foot back. Continue alternating the feet as fast as you can without sacrificing form.

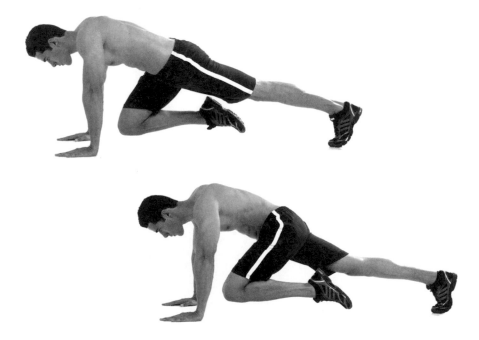

Right-Left Punch

level 3

 Stand with left foot forward in a fighting stance, fists up.

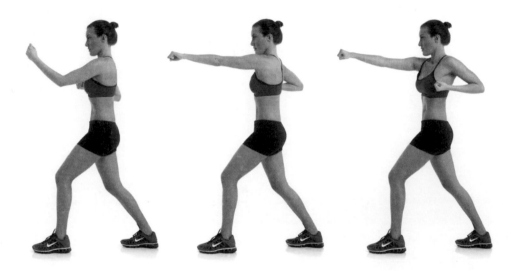

 Pivot your right hip forward, extending and jabbing with the right arm. Your fist should be parallel to the floor at full extension, and your arm should stay in line with your shoulder.

 Recoil immediately and punch with the left arm, pulling the right arm back, close to the body. Repeat as fast as you can without sacrificing form, and switching legs at the 25-second mark.

Salmon Jump

level 3

 Stand with knees slightly bent. Jump forward and to the left at a diagonal, pushing off the outside of the foot.

 Without pausing, jump again, this time traveling forward and to the right. Be sure to land with knees bent.

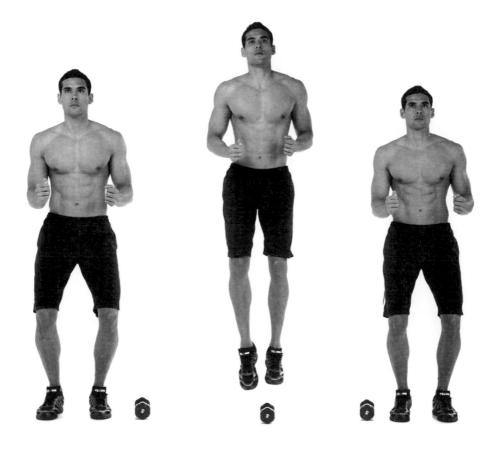

 Repeat 2 or 3 more times, jumping from side to side, until you have traveled about 10 feet forward. This is 1 complete rep. Then turn around and come back the other direction.

Back Kick

level 3

 Stand in fighting stance.

 Placing your weight on the front leg, lift the right knee. Then kick back through that leg, flexing your foot as if using the heel as a striking surface.

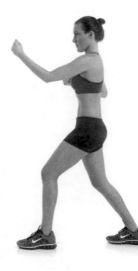

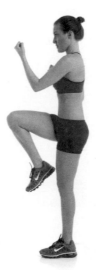

 Lower your leg back to the starting position. Do as many kicks with the right leg as you can. Switch to the left leg.

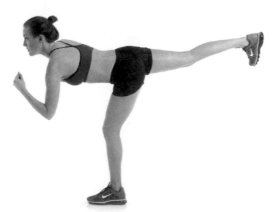

Burpees

level 3

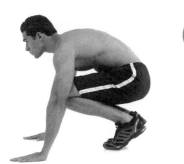

1 Begin standing. Drop into a squat position with hands on the floor in front of you.

2 Kick your feet back into a push-up position without letting your hips sag.

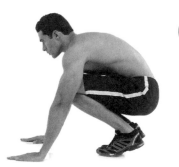

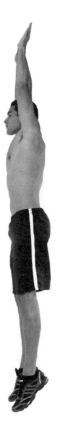

3 Immediately jump your feet back to the squat position.

4 Then jump straight up as high as you can for 1 complete rep.

Notes

Upper Body

These upper body exercises will work different parts of your chest, back, shoulders, as well as the upper and lower arms.

Challenge yourself, but don't sacrifice form. It's better to do fewer high-quality reps than a higher number of reps with bad form.

Bent Row

level 1

 Stand with feet shoulder-width apart, holding a dumbbell in each hand, palms facing your thighs. Hinge forward at the hips so your torso is parallel or almost parallel to the floor.

 Bend at the elbows, pulling arms straight back until weights are at chest-height. Squeeze the shoulder blades at the top of the row. Lower your arms for 1 rep.

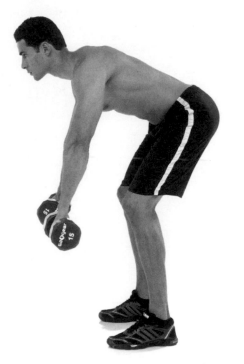

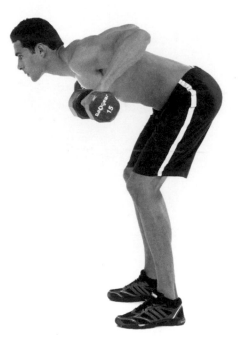

Chest Fly On Stability Ball

level 1

1 Lie in a table position with your shoulders and upper back on a stability ball, and feet on the floor hip-width apart. Hold a dumbbell in each hand above your chest, palms facing out. Keep your core engaged and your hips lifted.

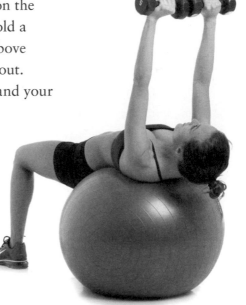

2 With slightly bent elbows, lower your arms down and back. Don't let arms go below chest-height. Press arms back up. Touch to complete 1 rep.

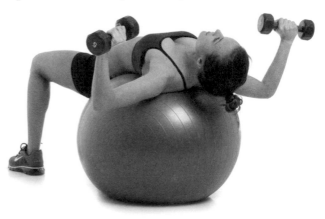

Tricep Kickbacks

level 1

 Stand with feet shoulder-width apart, holding a dumbbell in each hand, palms facing your sides. Hinge forward at the hips so your torso is parallel or almost parallel to the floor. Bend at the elbow in a 45-degree angle and pull up your right arm, so the upper arm is parallel to the floor.

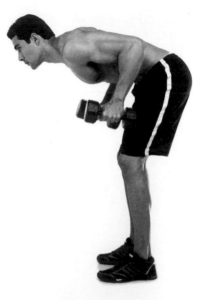

 Keeping your right upper arm still, raise your forearm so the weight stretches out behind you and your arm is straight, squeezing the tricep and upper back. Reverse the motion for 1 rep. Repeat as many times as you can, switching arms at the 25-second mark.

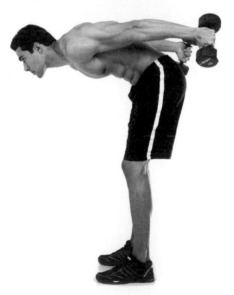

Bicep Curl

level 1

 Stand with your feet shoulder-width apart, holding a dumbbell in each hand, palms facing up.

 Curl both dumbbells up in a slow, controlled motion, keeping the arms close to the sides of the body. Lower to starting position and repeat. If this exercise is too difficult, you can curl one arm at a time.

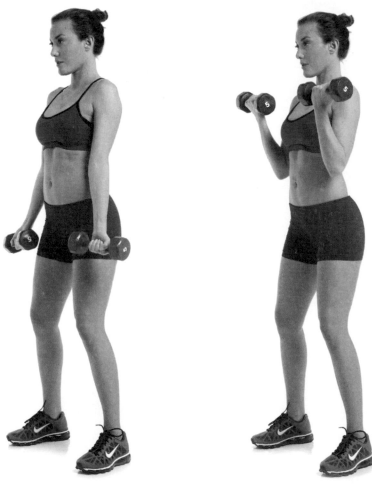

Modified Push-ups

level 1

 Get into a traditional push-up position but put your knees on the ground with feet crossed at ankles.

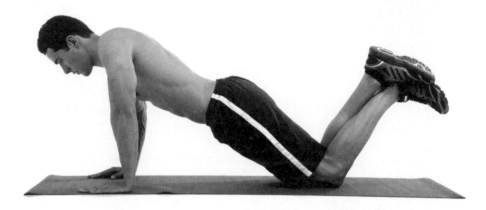

 Lower toward the ground without letting your hips sag, keeping your body in a straight line from head to knees.

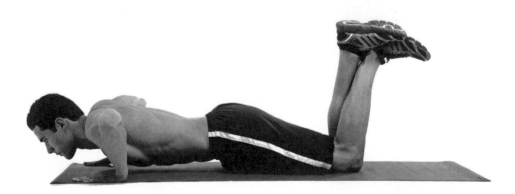

Close Chest Press on Ball

level 1

1 Lie back so your feet are on the floor about hip-width apart, and your upper back is resting on a stability ball, forming a table position. Hold a set of dumbbells directly over your chest, palms facing each other, with the dumbbells touching.

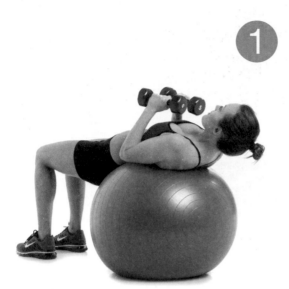

2 Lower the set of dumbbells to the center of your chest. Then press them back up to the starting position for 1 rep. If this exercise is too difficult, you can alternate arms one at a time.

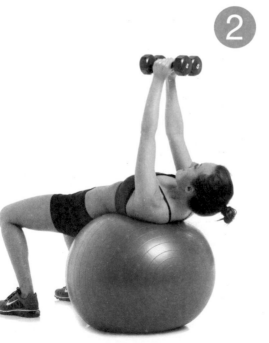

Push-ups

level 2

 Get into a traditional push-up position with straight arms and legs, body lifted off the floor. Keep your toes tucked under your feet, and arms under shoulders.

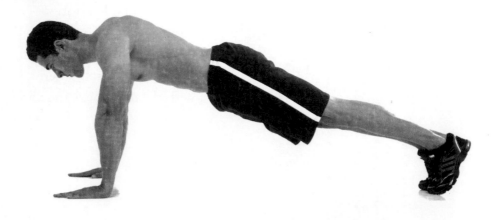

 Bend your arms and lower your body to the floor. Do not arch your back or let your hips sag. Push back up and straighten your arms for 1 rep.

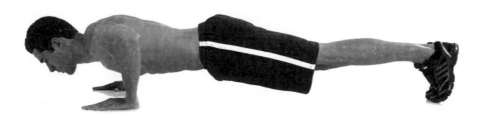

Seated Tricep Extensions

level 2

 Sit on a stability ball, holding a dumbbell at one end in both hands, with hands overlapping one another. Then extend the arms overhead by the ears.

 Lower the dumbbell behind your head until arms reach about a 90-degree angle. Then press the arms back up to straighten. Keep the core engaged to avoid arching your back.

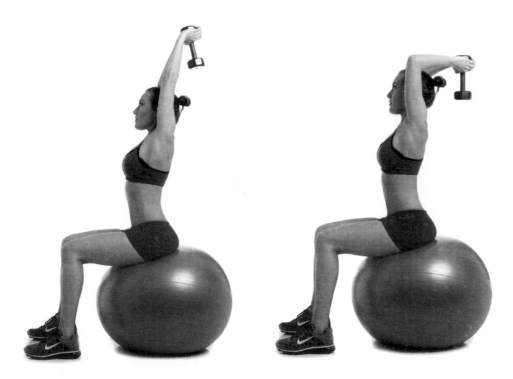

Y Raise & Shrug

level 2

 Stand holding a pair of dumbbells at your side, palms facing inward.

 Raise your arms up and slightly out so they form a Y shape. Lift them until they are parallel to the floor and level with your shoulders.

 Pause at the top of the movement and shrug your shoulders up toward your ears. Pause for another second, then lower the arms back to your sides for 1 rep.

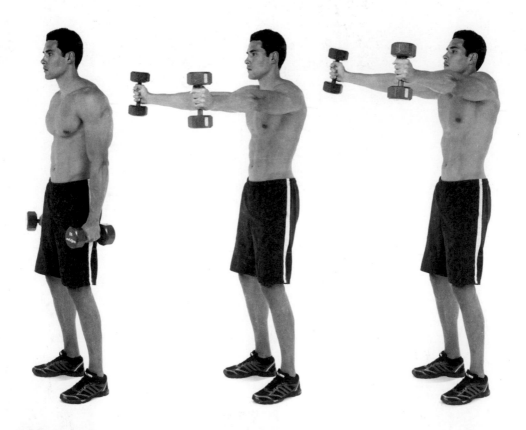

Front Raise

level 2

 Hold a pair of dumbbells with an overhand grip, palms facing back. Let arms hang down by your sides. Feet should be shoulder-width apart.

2 Raise your arms straight out in front of you until they're parallel to the floor and in line with your shoulders. Pause for a second, then lower back to the starting position.

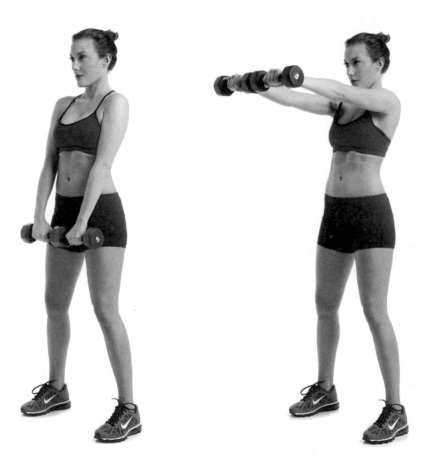

Rear Lateral Raise

level 2

 Hold a pair of dumbbells in both hands. Keeping a slight bend in your knees, bend forward so your torso is almost parallel to the floor. Hold your arms straight down in front of you, with palms facing each other.

 Keeping a slight bend in the elbows and your torso, lift your arms straight up and out to the sides until they become even with your shoulders. Squeeze your upper back between your shoulders, then lower arms to the starting position.

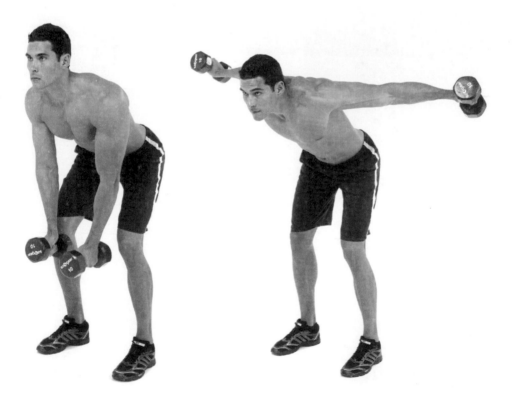

L Raise on Ball

level 2

 1 Lie stomach-down on a stability ball. Hold a light dumbbell in each hand, and let your arms hang straight down, palms facing back.

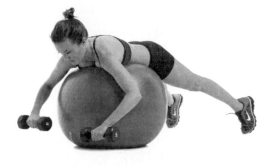

 2 Pull your elbows straight back and lift your upper arms until they are in line with the back. Your arms will form L shapes.

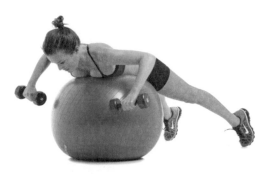

 3 Without moving your elbows, rotate your upper arms up and back, squeezing between the shoulder blades. Lower to the starting position and repeat.

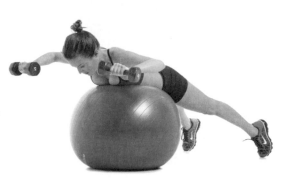

Lawn Mower

level 3

1 Bend forward at the waist so your torso forms nearly a 45-degree angle with the floor. Hold one dumbbell in your right hand, palm facing in, and your arm straight down.

2 Pull the dumbbell up toward your chest and rotate out to the right, twisting your torso up (imagine pulling a weed out of the ground). Lower back to the starting position and repeat, switching the dumbbell to the other hand at the 25-second mark.

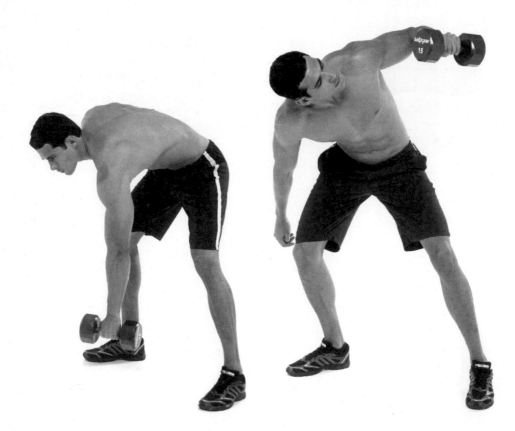

Dumbbell Swing

level 3

 Hold a dumbbell with an overhand grip (palm facing toward the body) between your legs. Bend your knees and squat down.

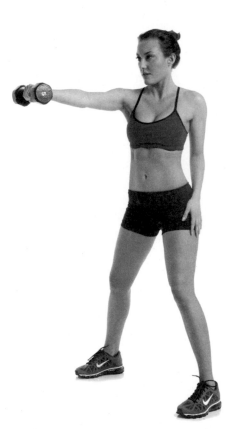 Thrusting through your glutes and hips, and squeezing the shoulders, stand up and swing the dumbbell up until it is chest-high.

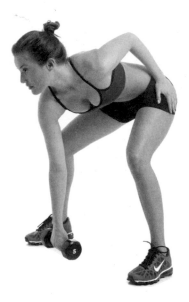

 Squat back down and swing the dumbbell back between your legs. Continue swinging the dumbbell back and forth fluidly and without sacrificing form. Switch arms at the 25-second mark.

Tricep Kickback w/ Twist

level 3

1 Stand with feet shoulder-width apart, holding a dumbbell in each hand in an overhand grip, palms facing back. Hinge forward at the hips so your torso is parallel or almost parallel to the floor. Bend at the elbow in a 45-degree angle and pull up both arms, so the upper arms are parallel to the floor.

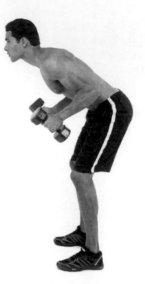

2 Keeping your upper arms still, extend your forearms so the weights stretch out behind you, palms facing the ceiling. Squeeze your upper back and tricep.

3 At the top of the movement, flip the weights in your hands so the palms face inward toward your sides. Then lower arms for 1 rep.

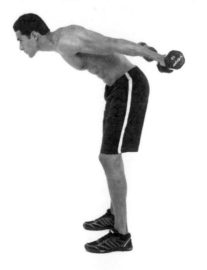

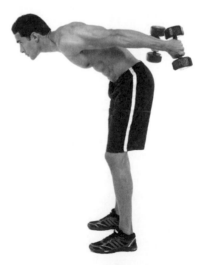

Judo Push-ups

level 3

1 Put your hands and feet flat on the ground with your hips lifted so your body forms an inverted V shape.

2 Keeping your hips up, bend your arms out to the side, and lower your upper body until your chin is near the floor.

3 Lower your hips toward the floor while you lift your upper body simultaneously. Then slide back into the original position, reversing the way you went in, for 1 rep.

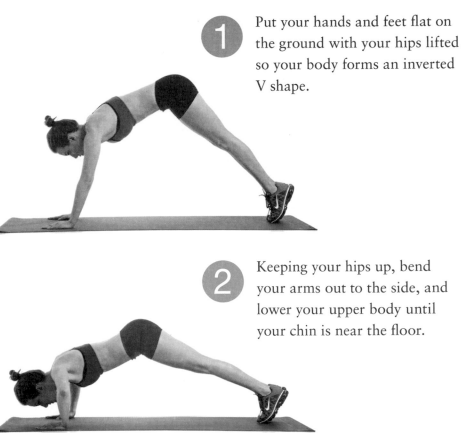

Shoulder Press w/ Twist

level 3

 Hold a pair of dumbbells up by your shoulders, with palms facing each other.

 Rotate your torso to the right and press the dumbbell in the left hand up above the shoulder.

 Reverse the motion. Rotate to the left side and press the right dumbbell up. Repeat, switching sides each time. Be sure to keep your abs tight and engaged.

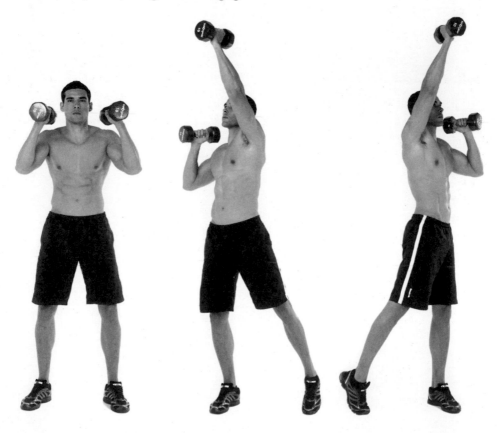

Bicep Curl to Overhead Press

level 3

 Stand holding a pair of dumbbells by your sides. Turning your palms so they're facing outward, curl the weights up, using the strength of your biceps.

 Fold your arms out so your elbows are at a 90-degree angle and upper arms are parallel to the floor.

 Press the weights up and over your head so the ends of the dumbbells touch or are in line. Don't forget to keep your shoulder blades back and your core engaged. Reverse the motion and return to the starting position.

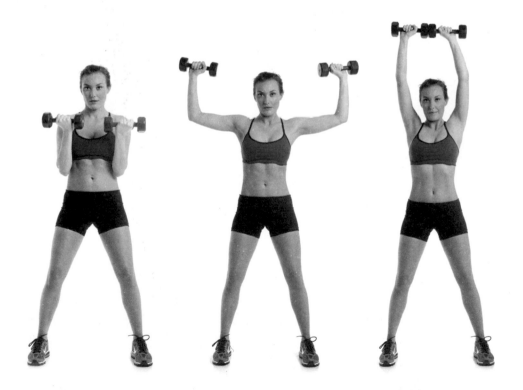

Notes

Ultra Simple 9-Minute Workouts

Exercise Plan

This section is your day by day exercise plan that will guide you through the next 9 weeks of workouts. Each day has two 9 minute workouts. One in the morning and one in the evening. Each workout is designed to target 1 of the 4 categories: core, lower body, cardio, and upper body. So, every day you will be working out different areas of your body.

This special exercise program is tiered into 3 levels. Level 1, makes up the first 3 weeks of the program. This level has beginning exercises that are not too difficult, yet are sure to get your whole body engaged and working. Level 2 builds on Level 1, and becomes more challenging. Weeks 4 through 6 will be harder than the previous 3 weeks, but not has challenging as the last 3 weeks. Level 3 contains the most difficult, but most rewarding exercises in the program.

LOOKING BACK

Take a moment to write about your current fitness level. Do you workout at all? If so, how many times a week and for how long? Be honest with yourself and describe how you feel about your current exercise regiment, as well as why you want to change. Also, write a commitment to yourself to stay focused and dedicated to the 9-Minute Workout Program.

DATE:_____   WEIGHT:_____

REFLECTION

DATE:_____   WEIGHT:_____

LOOKING FORWARD

Your expectations for Level 1:

_____

_____

_____

_____

_____

EXERCISE GOALS

Exercise goals for Level 1:

_____

_____

_____

_____

_____

_____

NOTES

Obstacles, solutions, and thoughts on your progress:

_____

_____

_____

_____

_____

_____

_____

_____

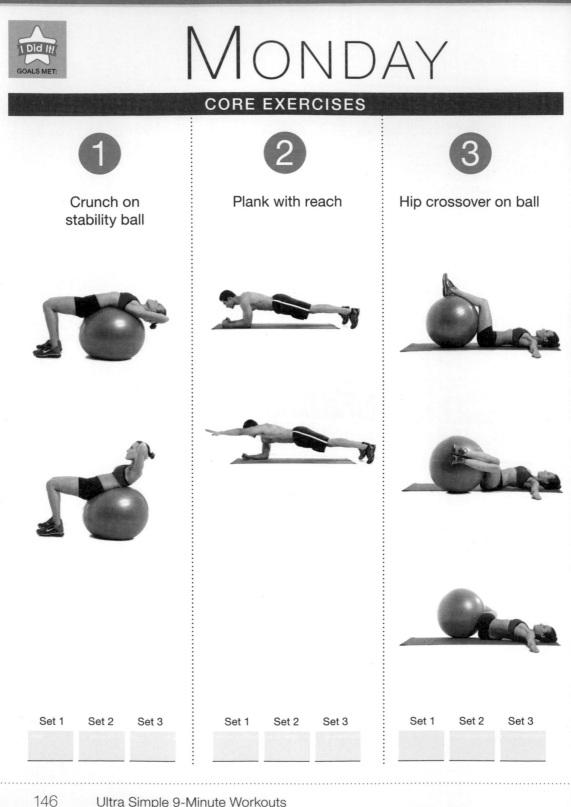

I Did It!

GOALS MET:

MONDAY

CORE EXERCISES

1
Crunch on stability ball

2
Plank with reach

3
Hip crossover on ball

Set 1	Set 2	Set 3

Set 1	Set 2	Set 3

Set 1	Set 2	Set 3

Week 1: Level 1

DATE:_____ WEIGHT:_____

LOWER BODY EXERCISES

1

Side leg raise with pulse

2

Fire hydrant

3

Body weight squat

Set 1	Set 2	Set 3

Set 1	Set 2	Set 3

Set 1	Set 2	Set 3

I Did It!
GOALS MET:

TUESDAY

CARDIO EXERCISES

1	**2**	**3**
Jog in place	Jumping jacks	Knee kick

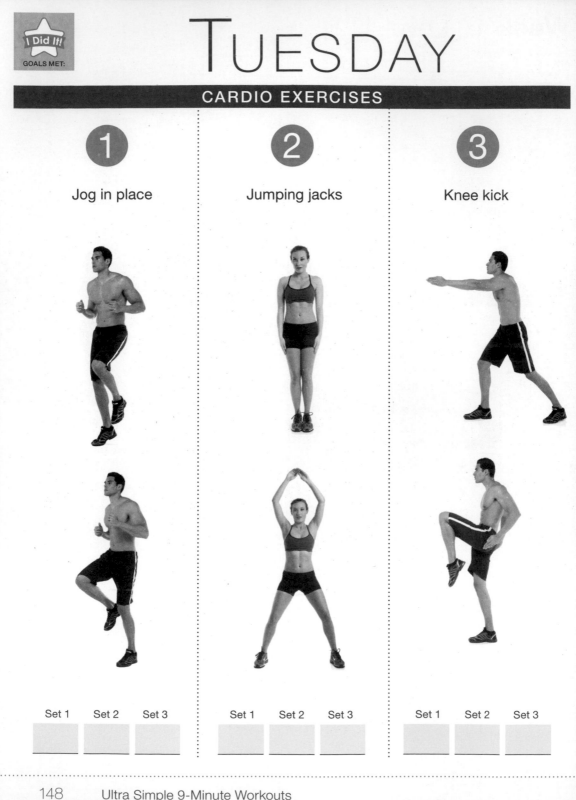

Set 1	Set 2	Set 3	Set 1	Set 2	Set 3	Set 1	Set 2	Set 3

Week 1: Level 1

DATE:_____   WEIGHT:_____

UPPER BODY EXERCISES

1

Chest fly on stability ball

2

Bent row

3

Bicep curl

Set 1	Set 2	Set 3

Set 1	Set 2	Set 3

Set 1	Set 2	Set 3

I Did It!
GOALS MET:

WEDNESDAY

CORE EXERCISES

1

Bird dog

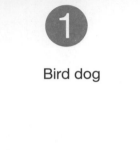

2

Side bend with dumbbell

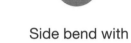

3

Beetle crunch

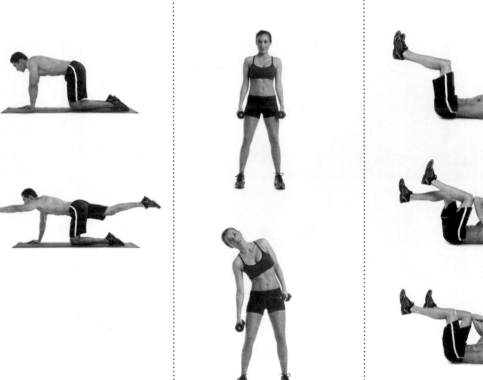

Set 1	Set 2	Set 3		Set 1	Set 2	Set 3		Set 1	Set 2	Set 3

Week 1: Level 1

DATE:_____ WEIGHT:_____

LOWER BODY EXERCISES

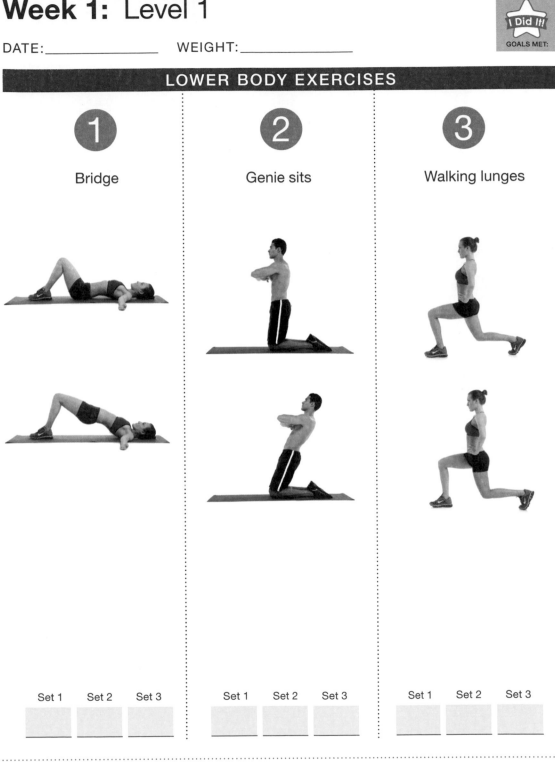

1

Bridge

2

Genie sits

3

Walking lunges

Set 1	Set 2	Set 3

Set 1	Set 2	Set 3

Set 1	Set 2	Set 3

I Did It!
GOALS MET:

THURSDAY

CARDIO EXERCISES

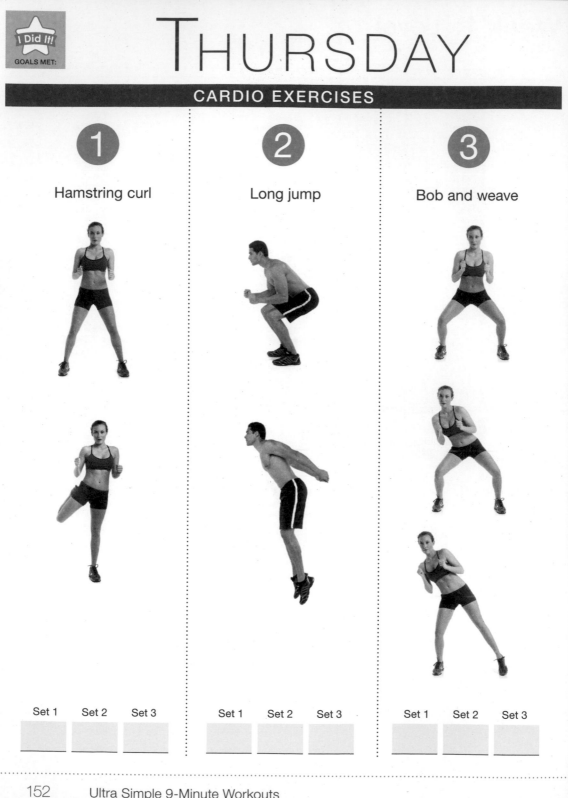

1

Hamstring curl

2

Long jump

3

Bob and weave

Set 1	Set 2	Set 3

Set 1	Set 2	Set 3

Set 1	Set 2	Set 3

Week 1: Level 1

DATE:_____ WEIGHT:_____

I Did It!

GOALS MET:

UPPER BODY EXERCISES

1

Tricep kickbacks

2

Close grip chest press on ball

3

Modified push-up

Set 1	Set 2	Set 3

Set 1	Set 2	Set 3

Set 1	Set 2	Set 3

I Did It!
GOALS MET:

FRIDAY

CORE EXERCISES

1

Plank with reach

2

Hip crossover on ball

3

Bird dog

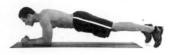

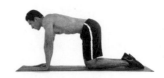

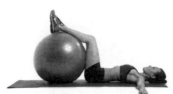

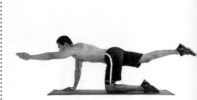

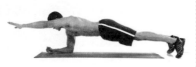

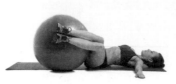

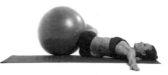

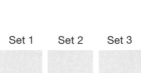

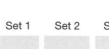

Set 1	Set 2	Set 3

Set 1	Set 2	Set 3

Set 1	Set 2	Set 3

Week 1: Level 1

DATE:_____   WEIGHT:_____

I Did It!
GOALS MET:

LOWER BODY EXERCISES

1
Fire hydrant

2
Body weight squat

3
Bridge

Set 1	Set 2	Set 3

Set 1	Set 2	Set 3

Set 1	Set 2	Set 3

I Did It!

GOALS MET:

SATURDAY

CARDIO EXERCISES

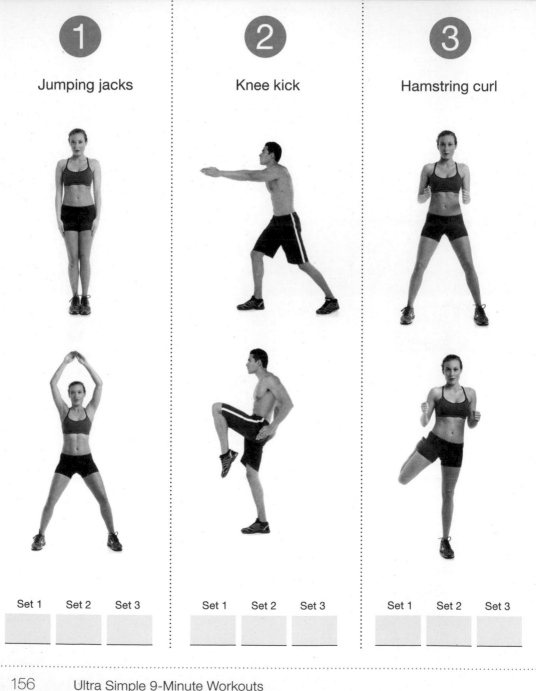

①	②	③
Jumping jacks	Knee kick	Hamstring curl

Set 1	Set 2	Set 3		Set 1	Set 2	Set 3		Set 1	Set 2	Set 3

Week 1: Level 1

DATE:_____   WEIGHT:_____

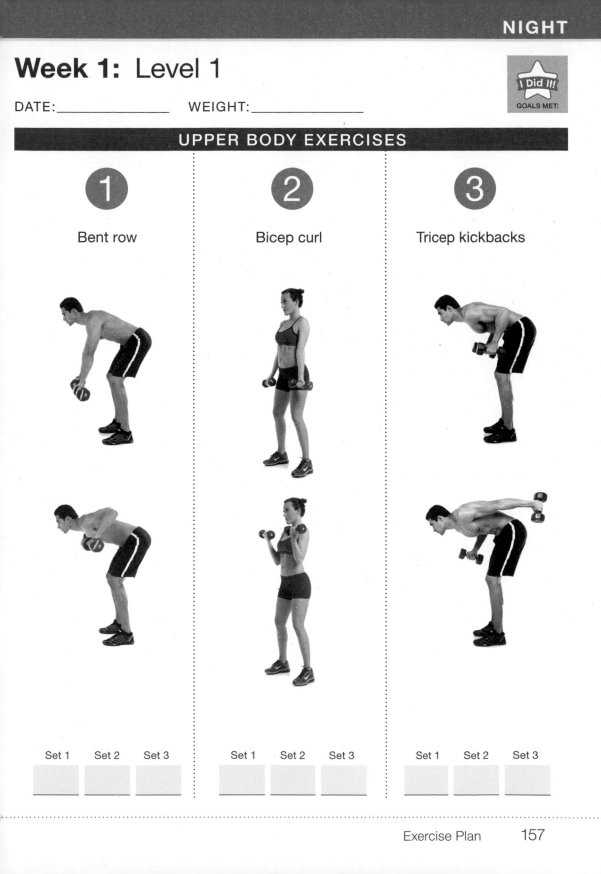

I Did It!
GOALS MET:

UPPER BODY EXERCISES

1

Bent row

2

Bicep curl

3

Tricep kickbacks

Set 1	Set 2	Set 3

Set 1	Set 2	Set 3

Set 1	Set 2	Set 3

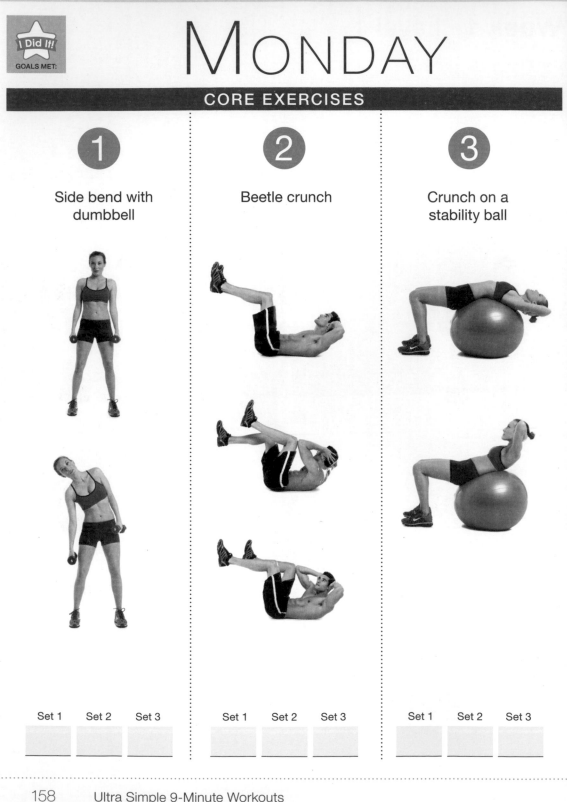

I Did It!
GOALS MET:

MONDAY

CORE EXERCISES

1

Side bend with dumbbell

2

Beetle crunch

3

Crunch on a stability ball

Set 1	Set 2	Set 3

Set 1	Set 2	Set 3

Set 1	Set 2	Set 3

Week 2: Level 1

DATE:_____   WEIGHT:_____

LOWER BODY EXERCISES

1	**2**	**3**
Genie sits	Walking lunges	Side leg raise with pulse

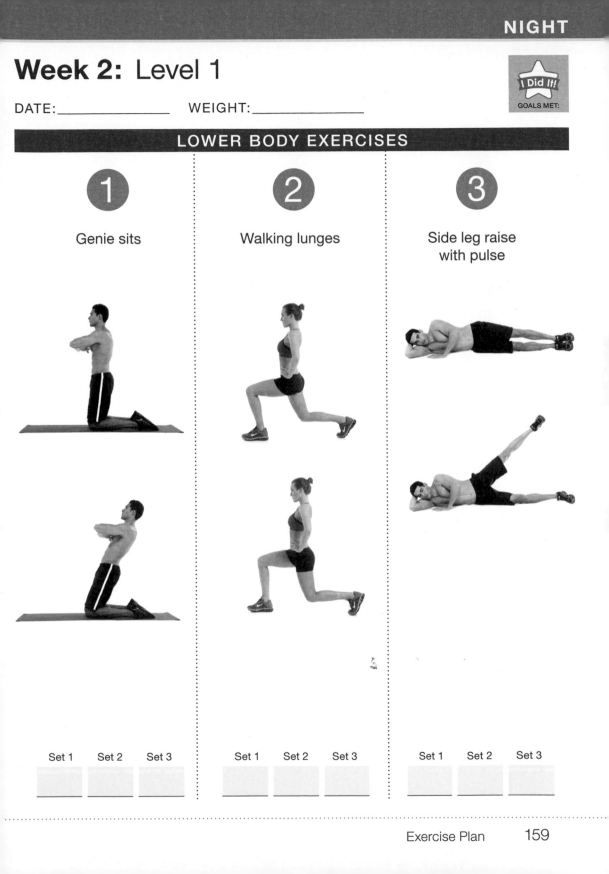

Set 1	Set 2	Set 3	Set 1	Set 2	Set 3	Set 1	Set 2	Set 3

TUESDAY

CARDIO EXERCISES

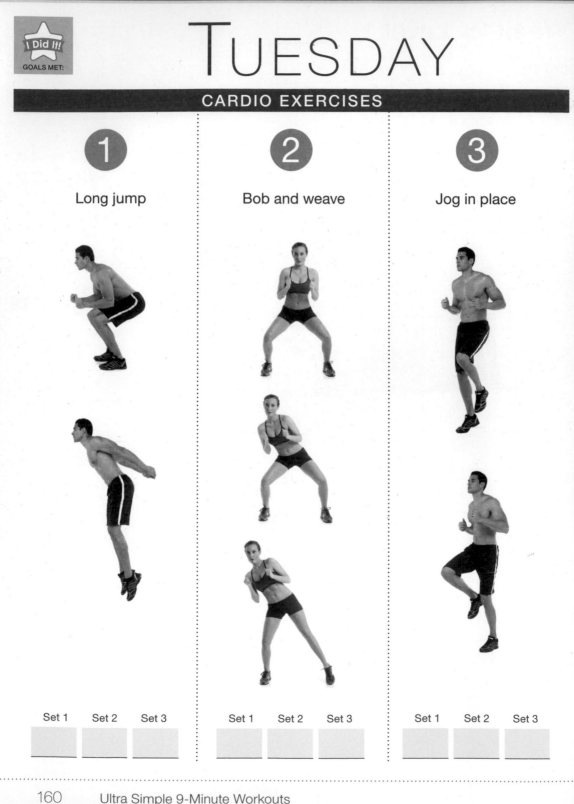

1 Long jump

2 Bob and weave

3 Jog in place

Set 1	Set 2	Set 3		Set 1	Set 2	Set 3		Set 1	Set 2	Set 3

Week 2: Level 1

DATE:_____   WEIGHT:_____

I Did It!
GOALS MET:

UPPER BODY EXERCISES

 1

 2

 3

| Close grip chest press on ball | Modified push-up | Chest fly on stability ball |

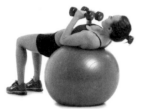

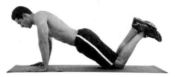

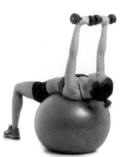

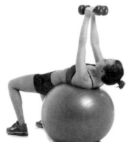

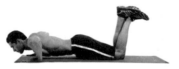

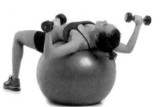

| Set 1 | Set 2 | Set 3 | Set 1 | Set 2 | Set 3 | Set 1 | Set 2 | Set 3 |

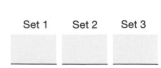

WEDNESDAY

CORE EXERCISES

1

Hip crossover on ball

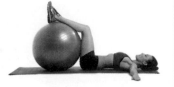

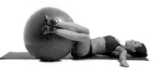

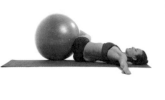

2

Bird dog

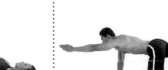

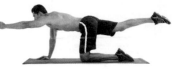

3

Side bend with dumbbell

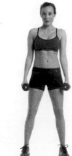

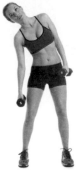

Set 1	Set 2	Set 3		Set 1	Set 2	Set 3		Set 1	Set 2	Set 3

Week 2: Level 1

DATE:_____   WEIGHT:_____

LOWER BODY EXERCISES

1

Body weight squat

2

Bridge

3

Genie sits

Set 1	Set 2	Set 3

Set 1	Set 2	Set 3

Set 1	Set 2	Set 3

THURSDAY

I Did It!
GOALS MET:

CARDIO EXERCISES

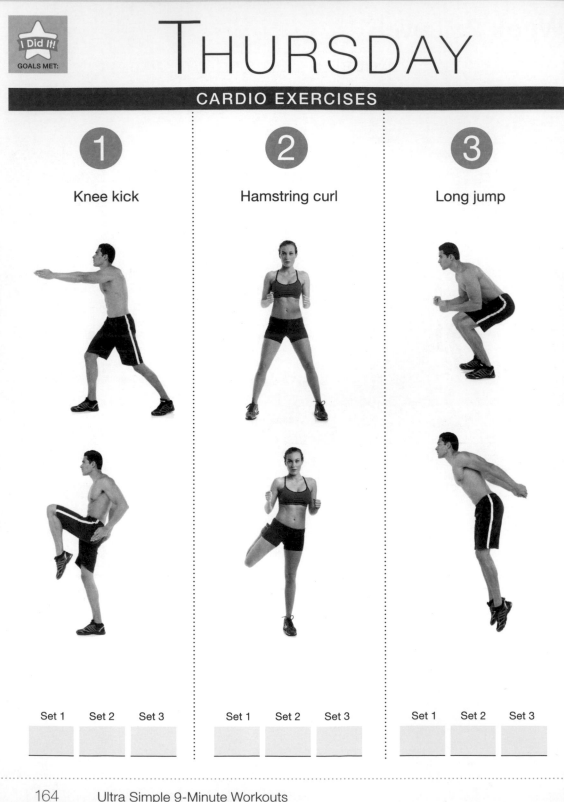

1 Knee kick

2 Hamstring curl

3 Long jump

Set 1 Set 2 Set 3

Set 1 Set 2 Set 3

Set 1 Set 2 Set 3

Week 2: Level 1

DATE:_____ WEIGHT:_____

UPPER BODY EXERCISES

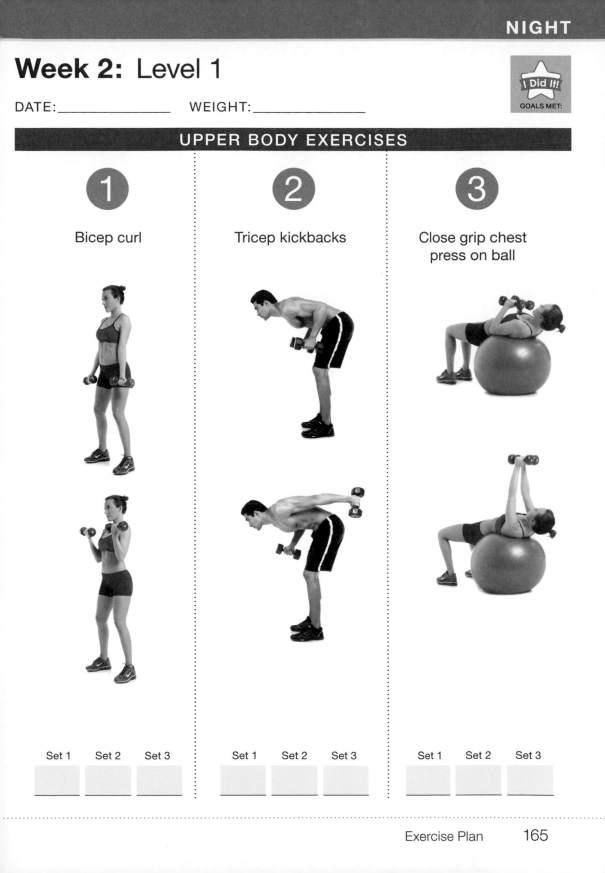

1 Bicep curl

2 Tricep kickbacks

3 Close grip chest press on ball

Set 1	Set 2	Set 3

Set 1	Set 2	Set 3

Set 1	Set 2	Set 3

FRIDAY

CORE EXERCISES

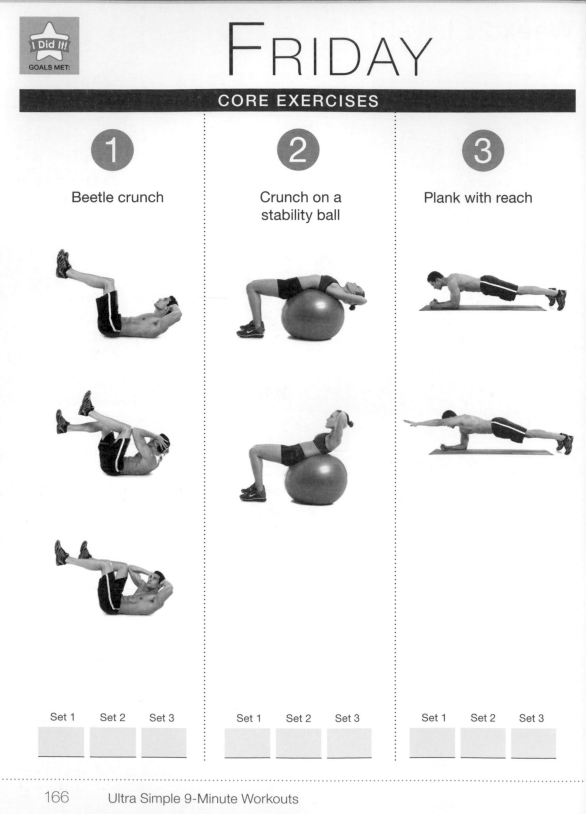

1 Beetle crunch

2 Crunch on a stability ball

3 Plank with reach

Set 1	Set 2	Set 3

Set 1	Set 2	Set 3

Set 1	Set 2	Set 3

I Did It! GOALS MET:

Week 2: Level 1

DATE:_____ WEIGHT:_____

I Did It!
GOALS MET:

LOWER BODY EXERCISES

Walking lunges

Side leg raise with pulse

Fire hydrant

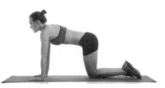

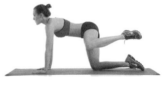

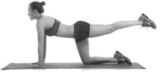

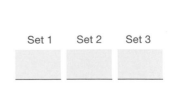

Set 1	Set 2	Set 3		Set 1	Set 2	Set 3		Set 1	Set 2	Set 3

I Did It!

GOALS MET:

SATURDAY

CARDIO EXERCISES

1 Bob and weave

2 Jog in place

3 Jumping jacks

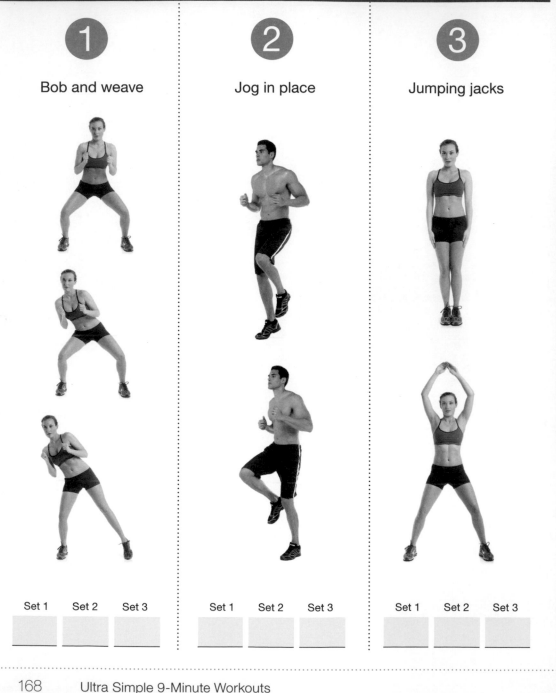

Set 1	Set 2	Set 3

Set 1	Set 2	Set 3

Set 1	Set 2	Set 3

Week 2: Level 1

DATE:_____   WEIGHT:_____

UPPER BODY EXERCISES

1

Modified push-up

2

Chest fly on
stability ball

3

Bent row

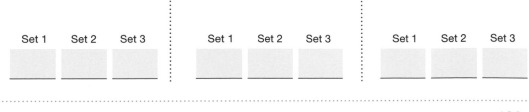

Set 1	Set 2	Set 3		Set 1	Set 2	Set 3		Set 1	Set 2	Set 3

I Did It!
GOALS MET:

MONDAY

CORE EXERCISES

1
2
3

Side bend with dumbbell

Bird dog

Crunch on a stability ball

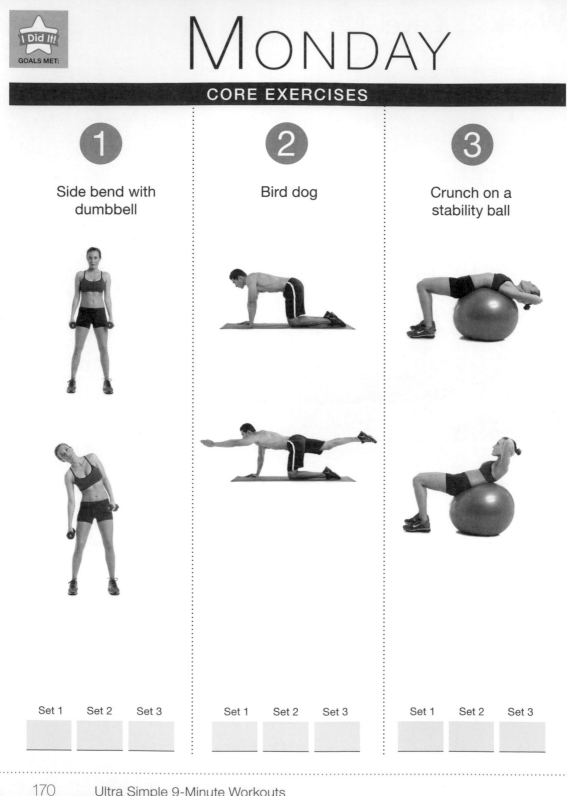

Set 1	Set 2	Set 3		Set 1	Set 2	Set 3		Set 1	Set 2	Set 3

Week 3: Level 1

DATE:_____   WEIGHT:_____

I Did It!
GOALS MET:

LOWER BODY EXERCISES

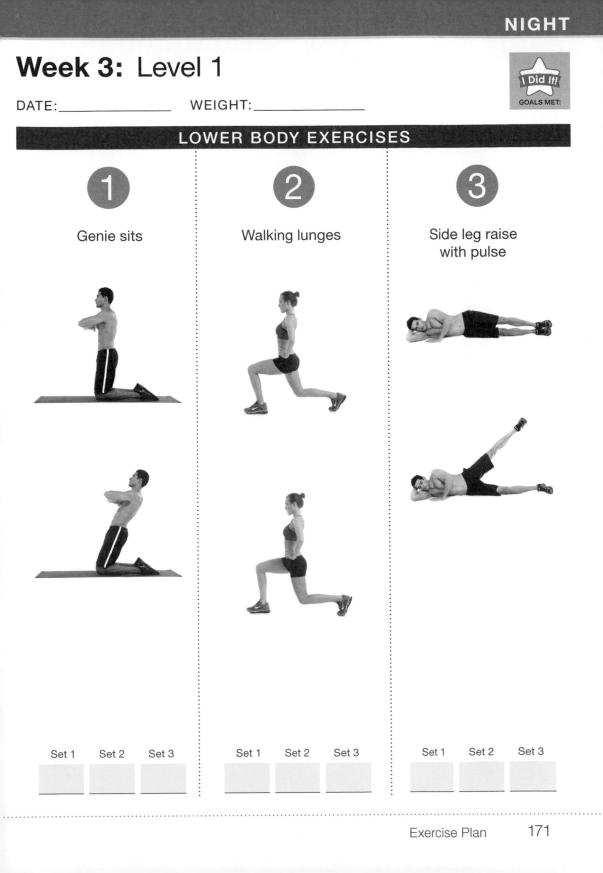

1	2	3
Genie sits	Walking lunges	Side leg raise with pulse

Set 1	Set 2	Set 3	Set 1	Set 2	Set 3	Set 1	Set 2	Set 3

I Did It!

GOALS MET:

TUESDAY

CARDIO EXERCISES

1	**2**	**3**
Long jump	Hamstring curl	Jog in place

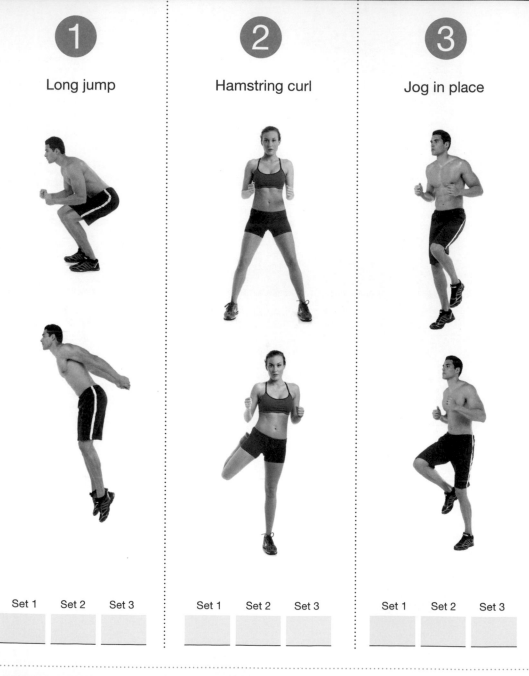

Set 1	Set 2	Set 3	Set 1	Set 2	Set 3	Set 1	Set 2	Set 3

Week 3: Level 1

DATE:_____   WEIGHT:_____

I Did It!
GOALS MET:

UPPER BODY EXERCISES

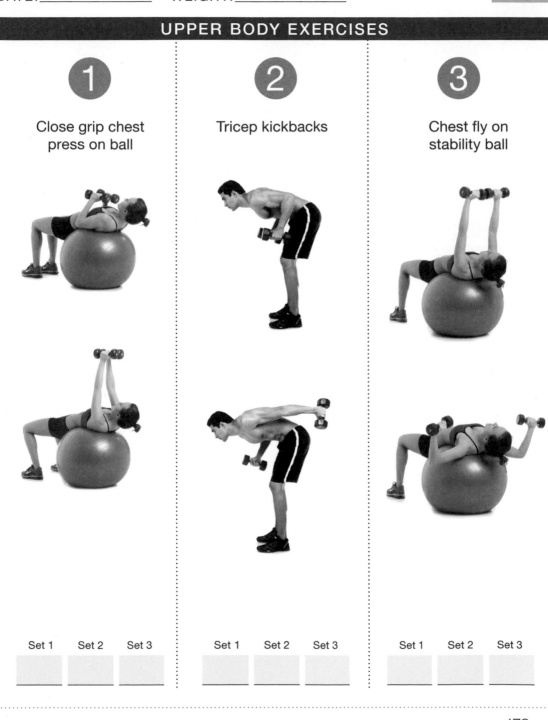

1
Close grip chest press on ball

2
Tricep kickbacks

3
Chest fly on stability ball

Set 1	Set 2	Set 3

Set 1	Set 2	Set 3

Set 1	Set 2	Set 3

GOALS MET:

WEDNESDAY

CORE EXERCISES

 1   **2**   **3**

Plank with reach	Hip crossover on ball	Beetle crunch

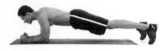

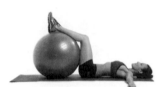

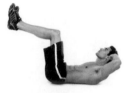

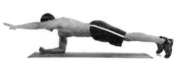

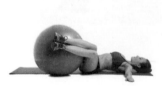

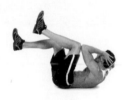

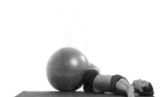

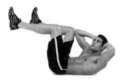

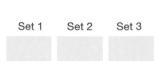

Set 1	Set 2	Set 3	Set 1	Set 2	Set 3	Set 1	Set 2	Set 3

Week 3: Level 1

DATE:_____ WEIGHT:_____

I Did It!
GOALS MET:

LOWER BODY EXERCISES

1

2

3

Fire hydrant

Body weight squat

Walking lunges

Set 1	Set 2	Set 3

Set 1	Set 2	Set 3

Set 1	Set 2	Set 3

THURSDAY

CARDIO EXERCISES

1	2	3
Jumping jacks	Knee kick	Bob and weave

I Did It!
GOALS MET:

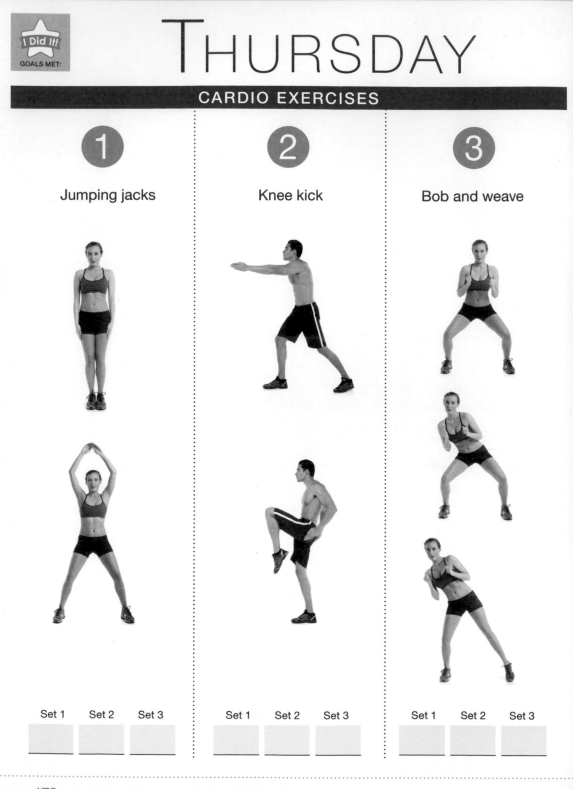

Set 1	Set 2	Set 3	Set 1	Set 2	Set 3	Set 1	Set 2	Set 3

Week 3: Level 1

DATE:_____   WEIGHT:_____

UPPER BODY EXERCISES

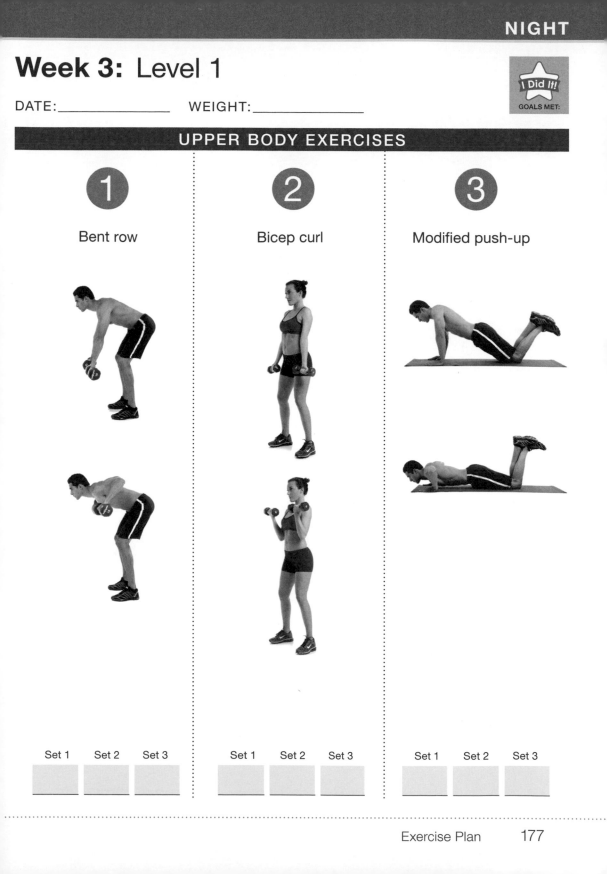

1

Bent row

2

Bicep curl

3

Modified push-up

Set 1   Set 2   Set 3

Set 1   Set 2   Set 3

Set 1   Set 2   Set 3

I Did It!
GOALS MET:

FRIDAY

CORE EXERCISES

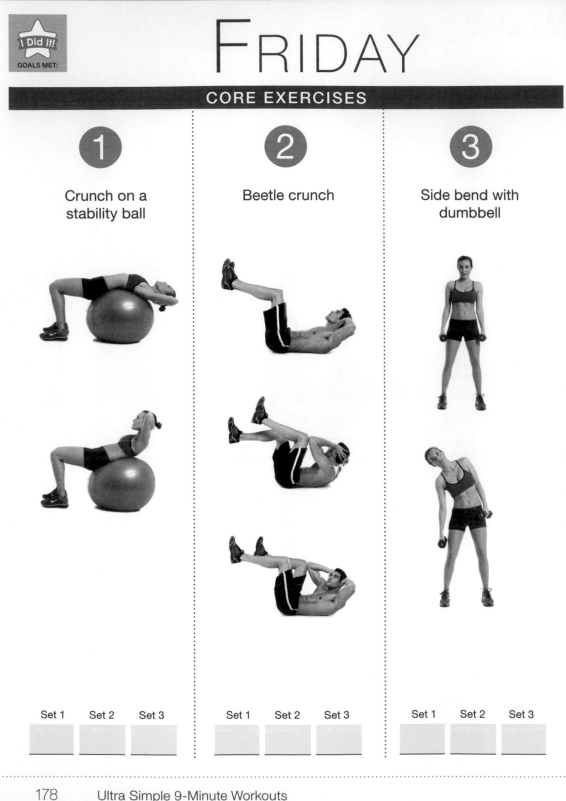

1

Crunch on a
stability ball

2

Beetle crunch

3

Side bend with
dumbbell

Set 1   Set 2   Set 3

Set 1   Set 2   Set 3

Set 1   Set 2   Set 3

Week 3: Level 1

DATE:_____   WEIGHT:_____

LOWER BODY EXERCISES

1

Side leg raise with pulse

2

Walking lunges

3

Genie sits

Set 1	Set 2	Set 3

Set 1	Set 2	Set 3

Set 1	Set 2	Set 3

SATURDAY

CARDIO EXERCISES

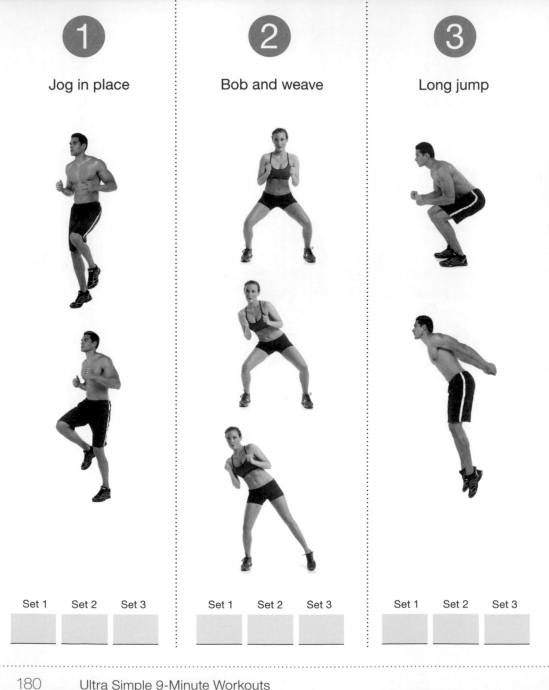

1	2	3
Jog in place	Bob and weave	Long jump

Set 1	Set 2	Set 3	Set 1	Set 2	Set 3	Set 1	Set 2	Set 3

Week 3: Level 1

DATE:_____ WEIGHT:_____

UPPER BODY EXERCISES

1

Chest fly on
stability ball

2

Modified push-up

3

Close grip chest
press on ball

Set 1	Set 2	Set 3

Set 1	Set 2	Set 3

Set 1	Set 2	Set 3

LOOKING BACK

DAYS I EXERCISED:

							WEEKLY ENERGY LEVEL:
Week 1:	☐ Mon. ☐ Tues. ☐ Wed. ☐ Thurs. ☐ Fri. ☐ Sat.						♡ low medium high ♡
Week 2:	☐ Mon. ☐ Tues. ☐ Wed. ☐ Thurs. ☐ Fri. ☐ Sat.						♡ low medium high ♡
Week 3:	☐ Mon. ☐ Tues. ☐ Wed. ☐ Thurs. ☐ Fri. ☐ Sat.						♡ low medium high ♡

LEVEL 1 HIGHLIGHT

Your greatest moment from Level 1:

_____

_____

_____

_____

_____

_____

EXERCISE GOALS

Did you meet your Level 1 goals?

_____

_____

_____

_____

_____

_____

IMPROVEMENTS

Ways to improve in the next level:

_____

_____

_____

_____

_____

_____

_____

DATE:_____   WEIGHT:_____

LOOKING FORWARD

Your expectations for Level 2:

_____

_____

_____

_____

_____

_____

EXERCISE GOALS

Exercise goals for Level 2:

_____

_____

_____

_____

_____

_____

_____

NOTES

Obstacles, solutions, and thoughts on your progress:

_____

_____

_____

_____

_____

_____

_____

_____

MONDAY

CORE EXERCISES

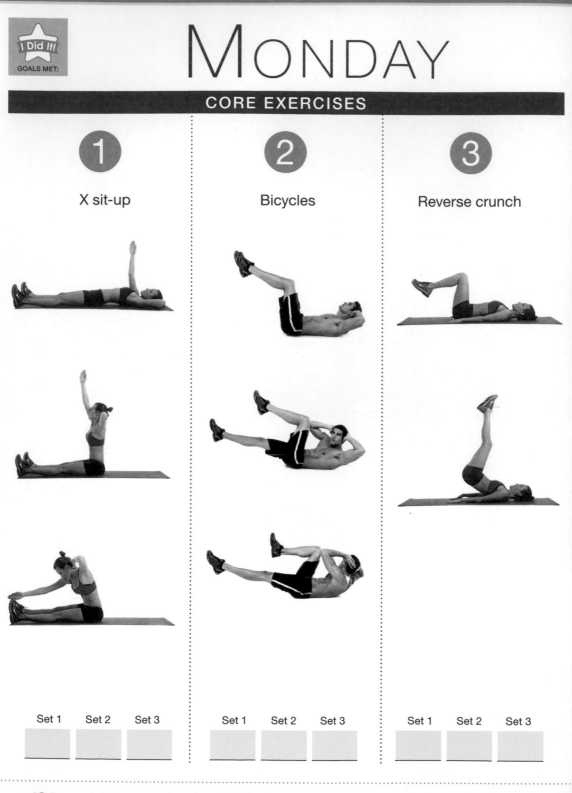

1 X sit-up

2 Bicycles

3 Reverse crunch

Set 1	Set 2	Set 3

Set 1	Set 2	Set 3

Set 1	Set 2	Set 3

I Did It!
GOALS MET:

Week 4: Level 2

DATE:_____ WEIGHT:_____

LOWER BODY EXERCISES

1

Lunges with a twist

2

Arabesque with dumbbell twist

3

Plié squat with pulse

Set 1	Set 2	Set 3

Set 1	Set 2	Set 3

Set 1	Set 2	Set 3

I Did It!
GOALS MET:

TUESDAY

CORE EXERCISES

1 Front kick

2 High knees

3 4 corner jump

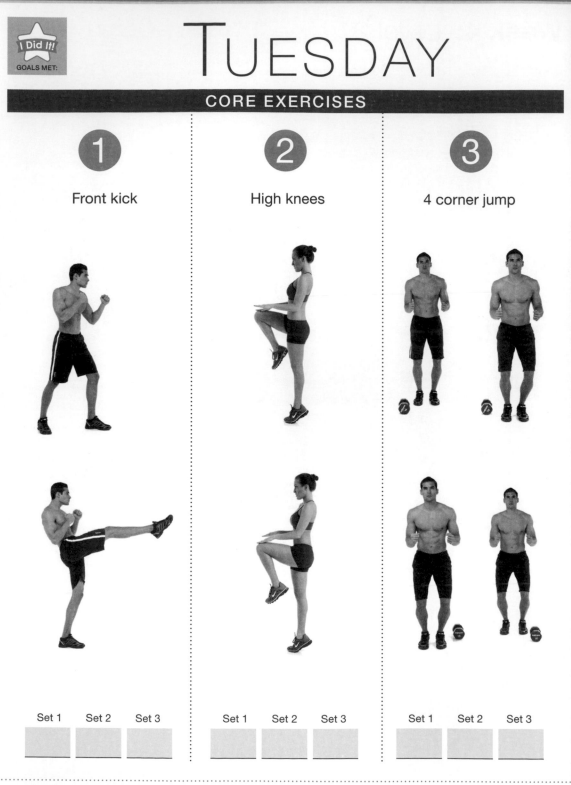

Set 1	Set 2	Set 3

Set 1	Set 2	Set 3

Set 1	Set 2	Set 3

Week 4: Level 2

DATE:_____ WEIGHT:_____

I Did It!
GOALS MET:

LOWER BODY EXERCISES

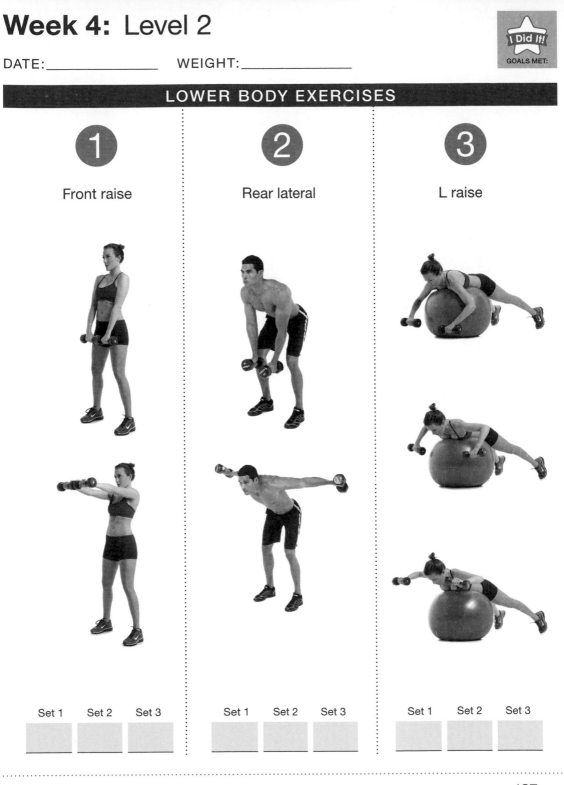

1 Front raise

2 Rear lateral

3 L raise

Set 1	Set 2	Set 3

Set 1	Set 2	Set 3

Set 1	Set 2	Set 3

WEDNESDAY

CORE EXERCISES

 1

Toe reach

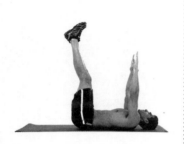

 2

Side plank with hip raise

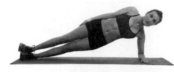

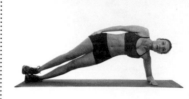

 3

Side crunch

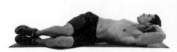

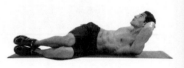

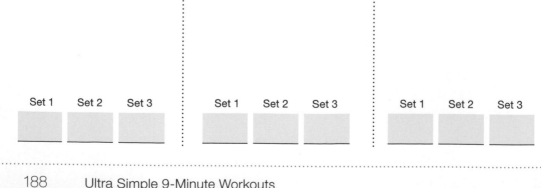

Set 1	Set 2	Set 3		Set 1	Set 2	Set 3		Set 1	Set 2	Set 3

Week 4: Level 2

DATE:_____ WEIGHT:_____

LOWER BODY EXERCISES

1

Single leg hip raise

2

Side lunge

3

Clamshell with dumbbell

Set 1	Set 2	Set 3

Set 1	Set 2	Set 3

Set 1	Set 2	Set 3

GOALS MET:

THURSDAY

CARDIO EXERCISES

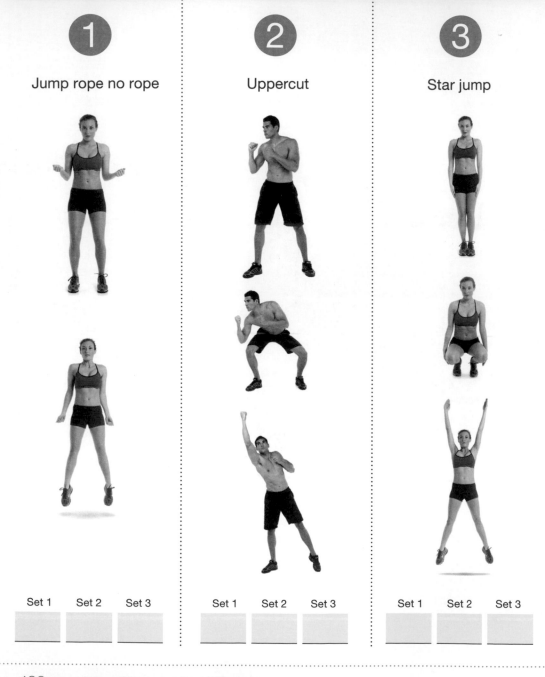

1

Jump rope no rope

2

Uppercut

3

Star jump

Set 1	Set 2	Set 3

Set 1	Set 2	Set 3

Set 1	Set 2	Set 3

Week 4: Level 2

DATE:_____   WEIGHT:_____

UPPER BODY EXERCISES

1

Push-up

2

Seated tricep extension

3

Y-front raise and shoulder shrug

Set 1	Set 2	Set 3

Set 1	Set 2	Set 3

Set 1	Set 2	Set 3

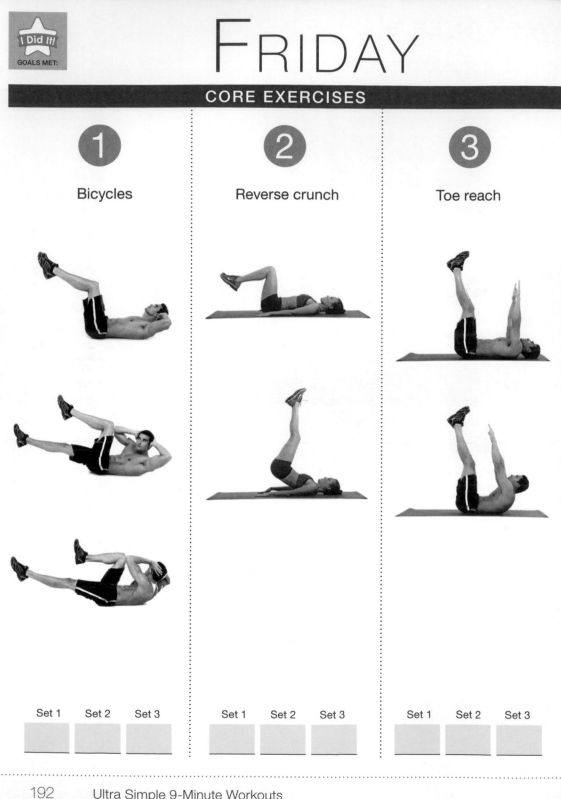

I Did It!

GOALS MET:

FRIDAY

CORE EXERCISES

1

Bicycles

2

Reverse crunch

3

Toe reach

Set 1	Set 2	Set 3

Set 1	Set 2	Set 3

Set 1	Set 2	Set 3

Week 4: Level 2

DATE:_____   WEIGHT:_____

LOWER BODY EXERCISES

1

Arabesque with dumbbell twist

2

Plié squat with pulse

3

Single leg hip raise

Set 1	Set 2	Set 3

Set 1	Set 2	Set 3

Set 1	Set 2	Set 3

I Did It!
GOALS MET:

SATURDAY

CARDIO EXERCISES

1 — High knees

2 — 4 corner jump

3 — Jump rope no rope

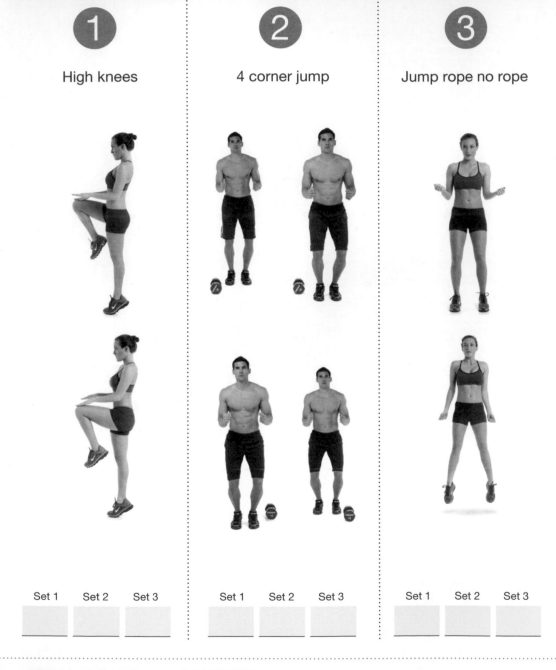

| Set 1 | Set 2 | Set 3 | | Set 1 | Set 2 | Set 3 | | Set 1 | Set 2 | Set 3 |

Week 4: Level 2

DATE:_____ WEIGHT:_____

UPPER BODY EXERCISES

1

Rear lateral

2

L raise

3

Push-up

Set 1	Set 2	Set 3

Set 1	Set 2	Set 3

Set 1	Set 2	Set 3

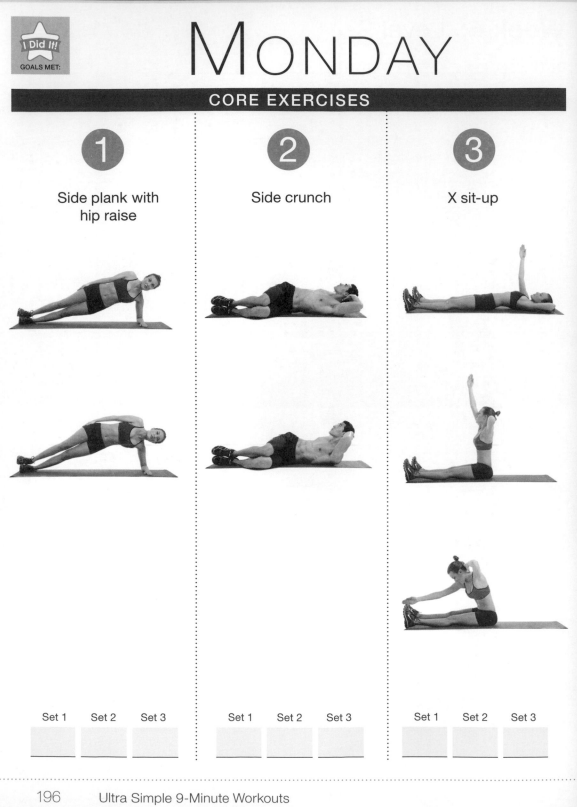

I Did It!
GOALS MET:

MONDAY

CORE EXERCISES

1
Side plank with hip raise

2
Side crunch

3
X sit-up

Set 1	Set 2	Set 3

Set 1	Set 2	Set 3

Set 1	Set 2	Set 3

Week 5: Level 2

DATE:_____ WEIGHT:_____

LOWER BODY EXERCISES

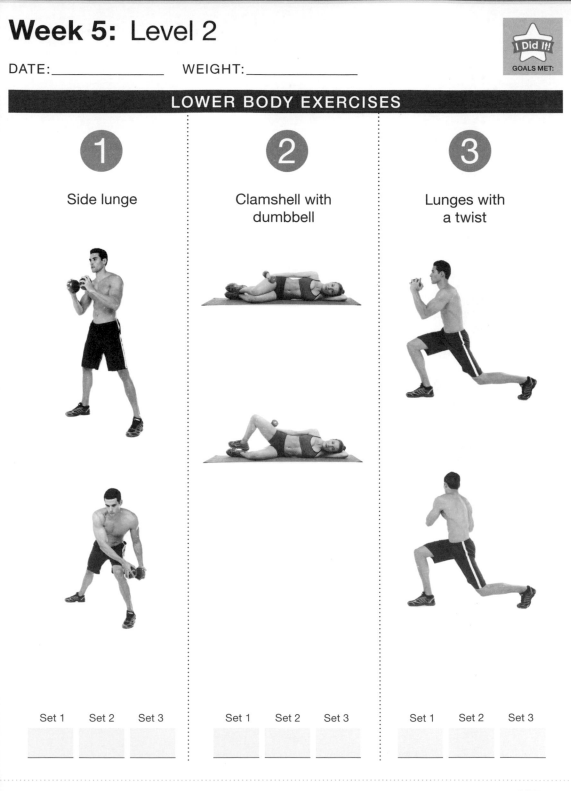

1

Side lunge

2

Clamshell with dumbbell

3

Lunges with a twist

Set 1	Set 2	Set 3

Set 1	Set 2	Set 3

Set 1	Set 2	Set 3

TUESDAY

I Did It! GOALS MET:

CARDIO EXERCISES

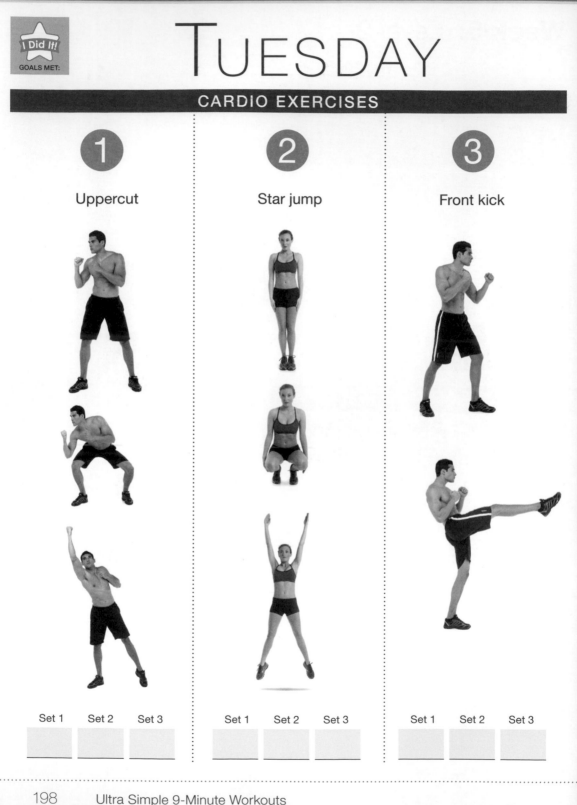

1

Uppercut

2

Star jump

3

Front kick

Set 1	Set 2	Set 3

Set 1	Set 2	Set 3

Set 1	Set 2	Set 3

Week 5: Level 2

DATE:_____ WEIGHT:_____

UPPER BODY EXERCISES

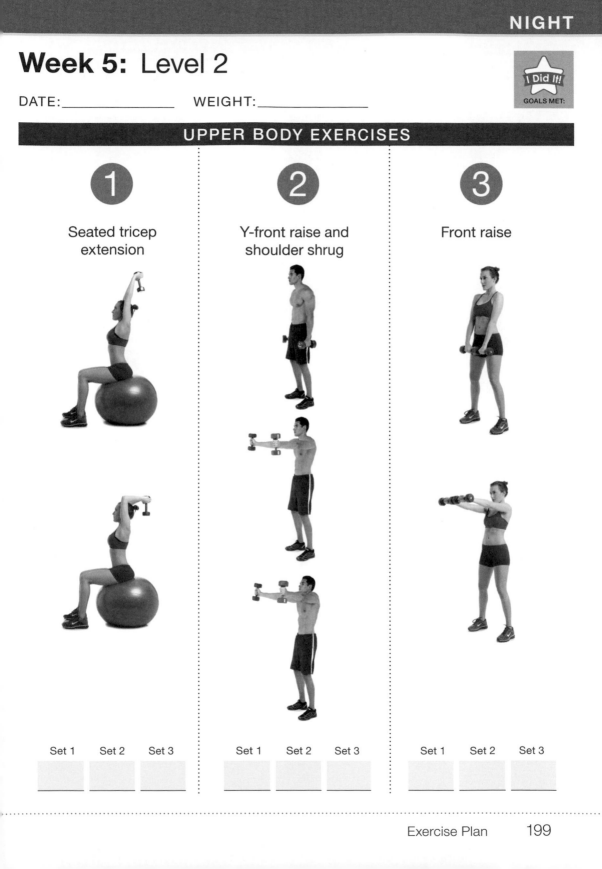

1

Seated tricep extension

2

Y-front raise and shoulder shrug

3

Front raise

Set 1	Set 2	Set 3		Set 1	Set 2	Set 3		Set 1	Set 2	Set 3

WEDNESDAY

CORE EXERCISES

1   **2**   **3**

Reverse crunch   Toe reach   Side plank with hip raise

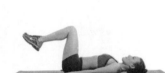 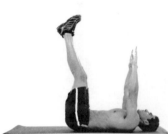 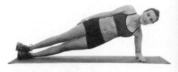

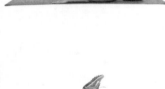 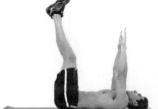

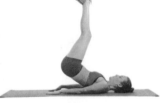 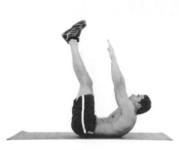 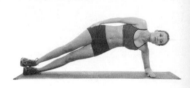

Set 1	Set 2	Set 3		Set 1	Set 2	Set 3		Set 1	Set 2	Set 3

Week 5: Level 2

DATE:_____   WEIGHT:_____

I Did It!
GOALS MET:

LOWER BODY EXERCISES

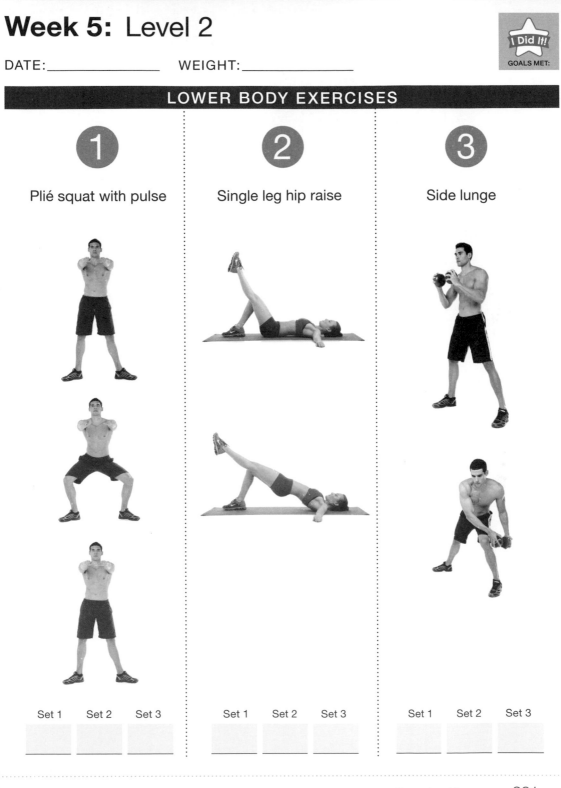

1 Plié squat with pulse

2 Single leg hip raise

3 Side lunge

Set 1	Set 2	Set 3

Set 1	Set 2	Set 3

Set 1	Set 2	Set 3

THURSDAY

I Did It!
GOALS MET:

CARDIO EXERCISES

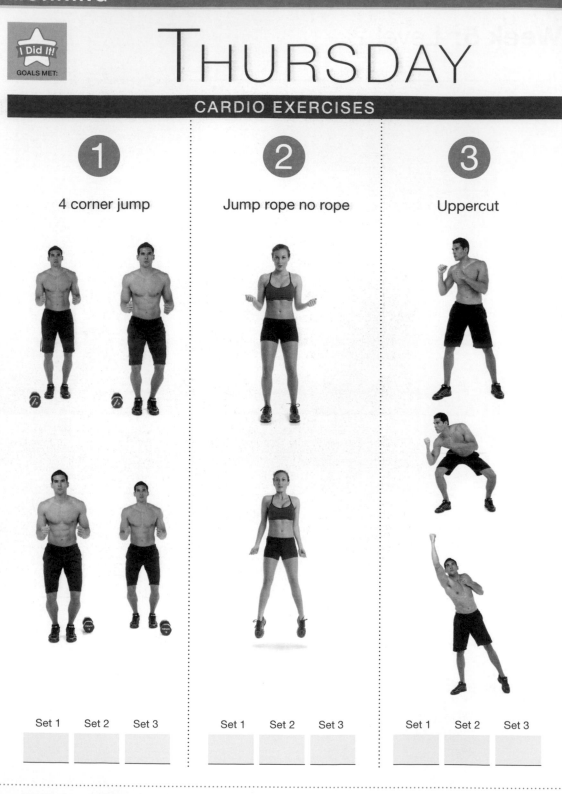

1 4 corner jump

2 Jump rope no rope

3 Uppercut

Set 1	Set 2	Set 3

Set 1	Set 2	Set 3

Set 1	Set 2	Set 3

Week 5: Level 2

DATE:_____   WEIGHT:_____

UPPER BODY EXERCISES

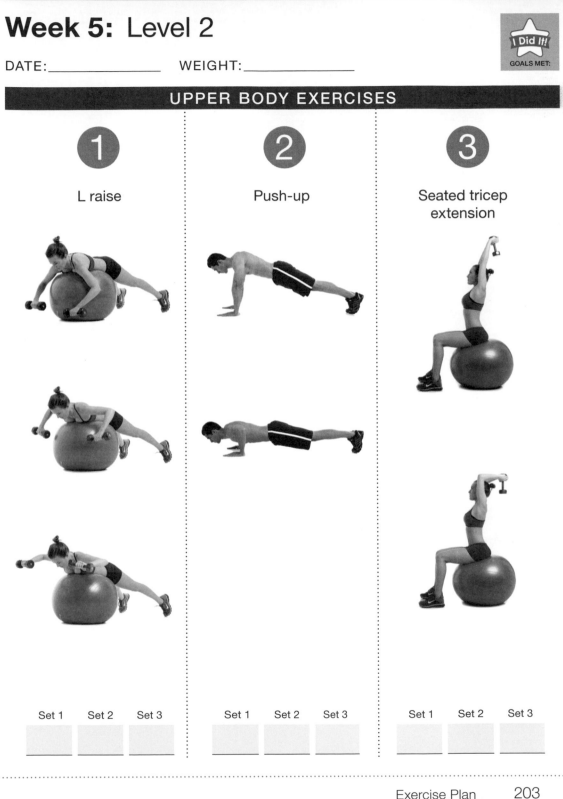

1 L raise

2 Push-up

3 Seated tricep extension

Set 1	Set 2	Set 3

Set 1	Set 2	Set 3

Set 1	Set 2	Set 3

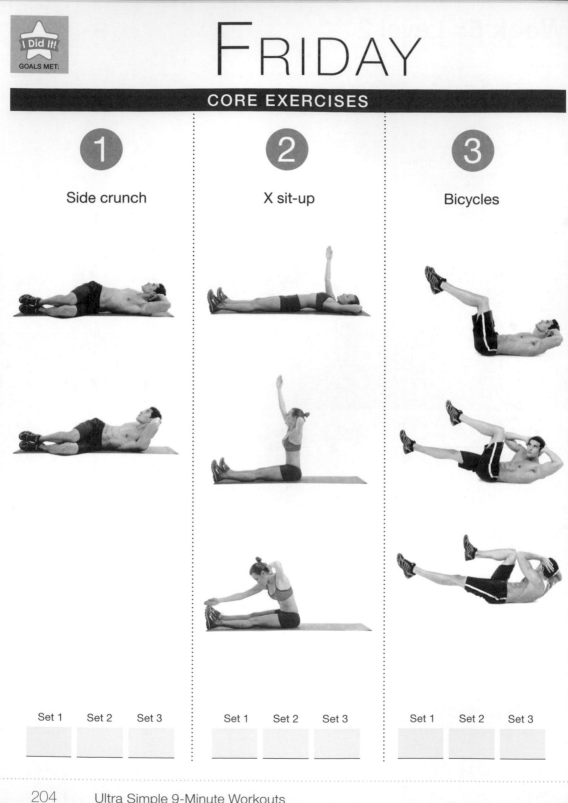

I Did It!
GOALS MET:

FRIDAY

CORE EXERCISES

1

Side crunch

2

X sit-up

3

Bicycles

Set 1 Set 2 Set 3

Set 1 Set 2 Set 3

Set 1 Set 2 Set 3

Week 5: Level 2

DATE:_____ WEIGHT:_____

I Did It!
GOALS MET:

LOWER BODY EXERCISES

1	2	3
Clamshell with dumbbell	Side lunge	Arabesque with dumbbell twist

Set 1	Set 2	Set 3		Set 1	Set 2	Set 3		Set 1	Set 2	Set 3

I Did It!
GOALS MET:

SATURDAY

CARDIO EXERCISES

1　Star jump

2　Front kick

3　High knees

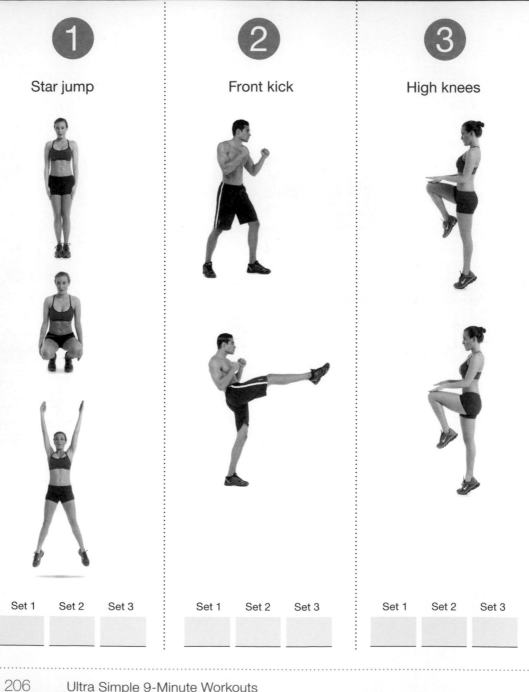

Set 1	Set 2	Set 3

Set 1	Set 2	Set 3

Set 1	Set 2	Set 3

Week 5: Level 2

DATE:_____   WEIGHT:_____

UPPER BODY EXERCISES

1

Y-front raise and shoulder shrug

2

Front raise

3

Rear lateral

| Set 1 | Set 2 | Set 3 | | Set 1 | Set 2 | Set 3 | | Set 1 | Set 2 | Set 3 |

I Did It!
GOALS MET:

MONDAY

CORE EXERCISES

1

Side plank with hip raise

2

Toe reach

3

X sit-up

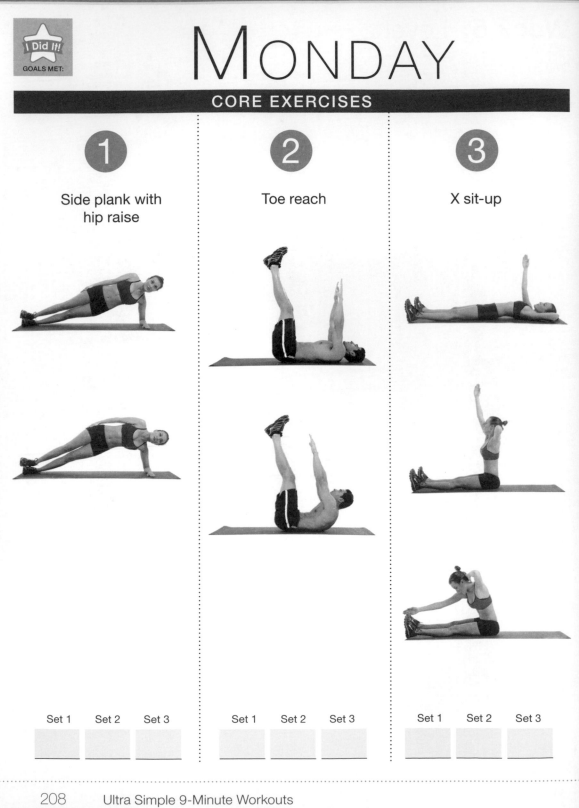

Set 1	Set 2	Set 3

Set 1	Set 2	Set 3

Set 1	Set 2	Set 3

Week 6: Level 2

DATE:_____   WEIGHT:_____

I Did It!
GOALS MET:

LOWER BODY EXERCISES

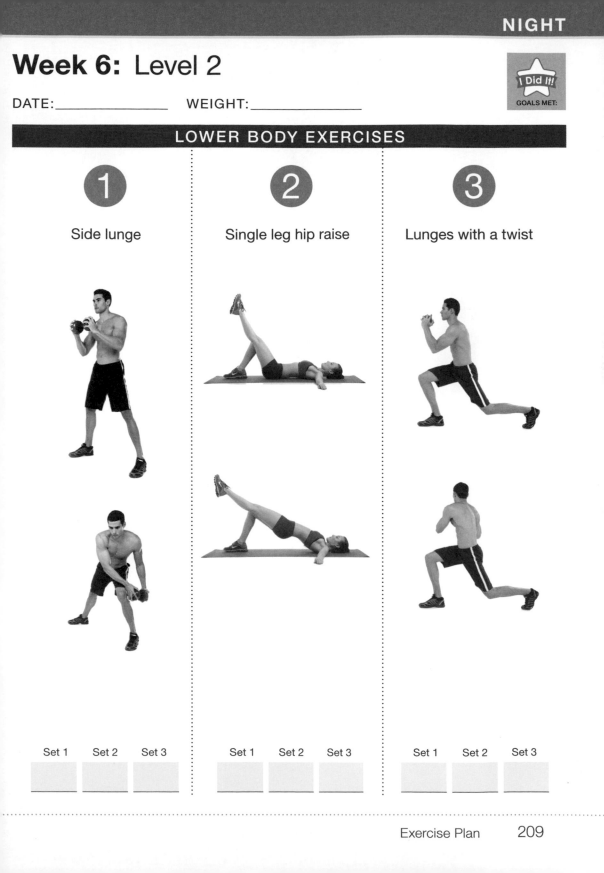

1

Side lunge

2

Single leg hip raise

3

Lunges with a twist

Set 1	Set 2	Set 3	Set 1	Set 2	Set 3	Set 1	Set 2	Set 3

GOALS MET:

TUESDAY

CARDIO EXERCISES

1	**2**	**3**
Uppercut	Jump rope no rope	Front kick

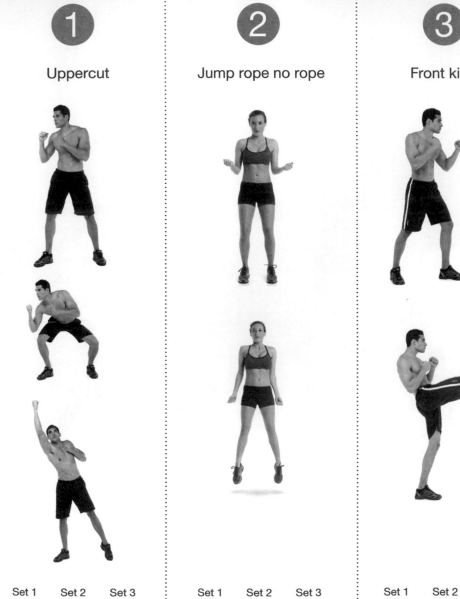

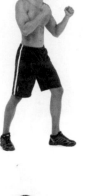

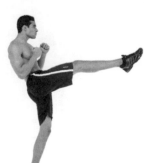

Set 1	Set 2	Set 3	Set 1	Set 2	Set 3	Set 1	Set 2	Set 3

Week 6: Level 2

DATE:_____ WEIGHT:_____

UPPER BODY EXERCISES

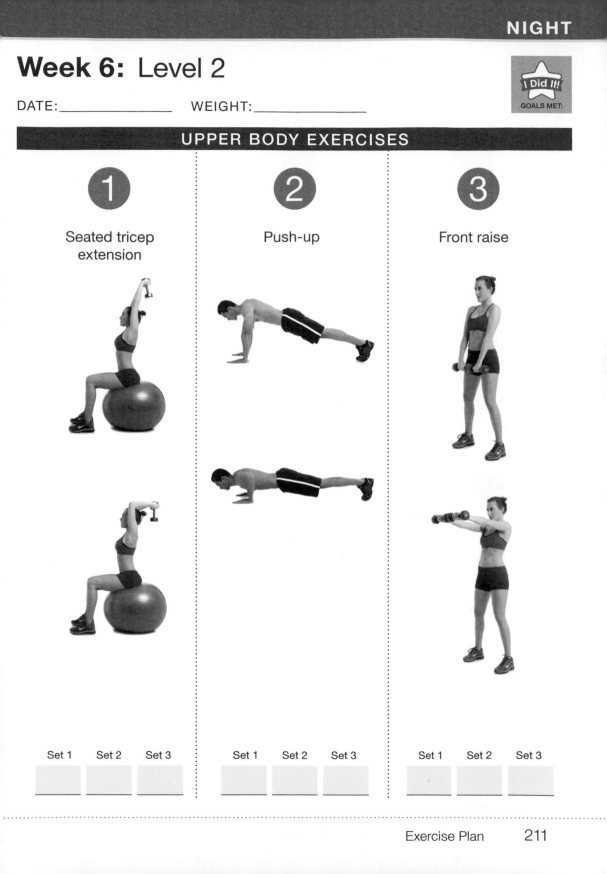

1 Seated tricep extension

2 Push-up

3 Front raise

Set 1	Set 2	Set 3

Set 1	Set 2	Set 3

Set 1	Set 2	Set 3

WEDNESDAY

CORE EXERCISES

 1

Bicycles

 2

Reverse crunch

 3

Side crunch

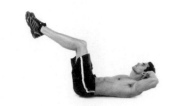

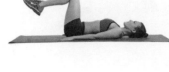

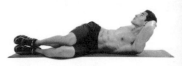

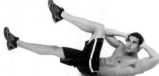

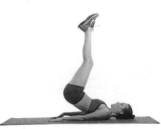

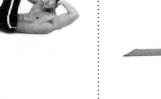

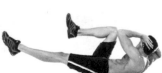

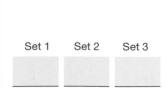

Set 1	Set 2	Set 3

Set 1	Set 2	Set 3

Set 1	Set 2	Set 3

Week 6: Level 2

DATE:_____   WEIGHT:_____

I Did It!
GOALS MET:

LOWER BODY EXERCISES

1

Arabesque with
dumbbell twist

2

Plié squat with pulse

3

Clamshell with
dumbbell

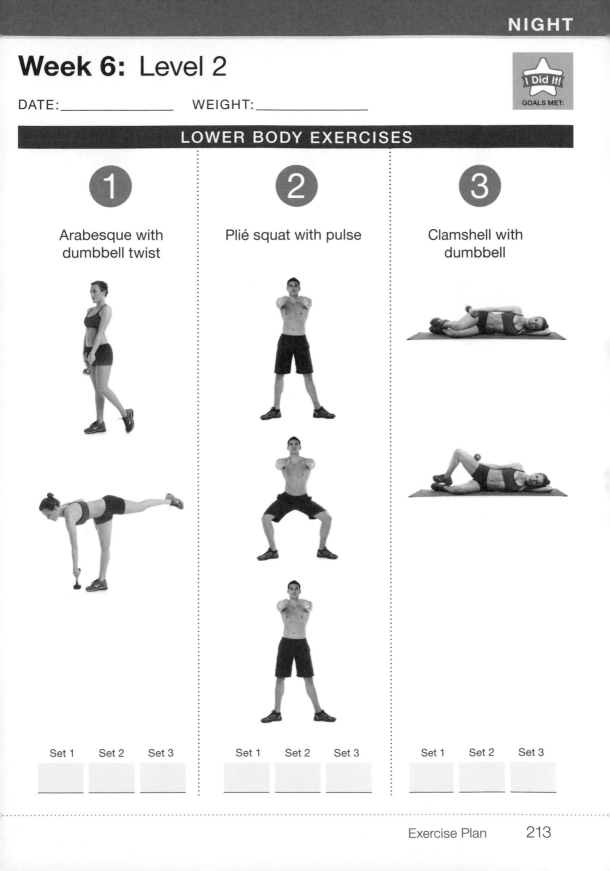

Set 1	Set 2	Set 3

Set 1	Set 2	Set 3

Set 1	Set 2	Set 3

CARDIO EXERCISES

1
High knees

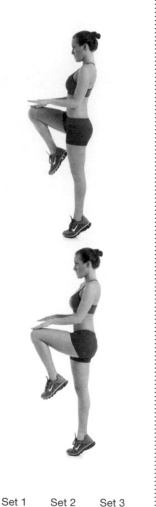

Set 1	Set 2	Set 3

2
4 corner jump

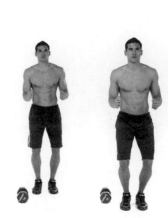
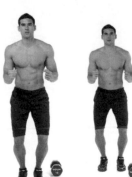
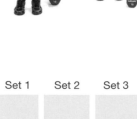

Set 1	Set 2	Set 3

3
Star jump

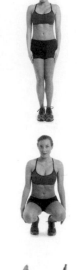
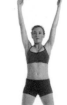

Set 1	Set 2	Set 3

Week 6: Level 2

DATE:_____ WEIGHT:_____

UPPER BODY EXERCISES

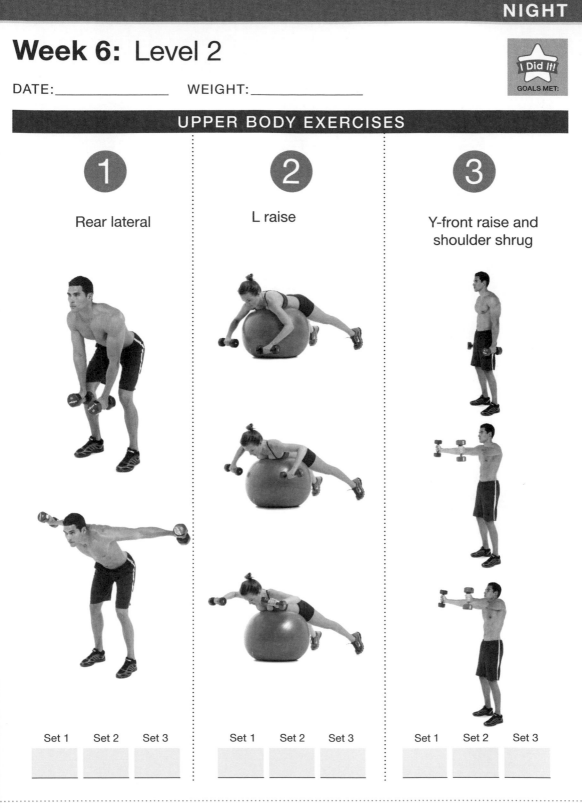

1

Rear lateral

2

L raise

3

Y-front raise and
shoulder shrug

Set 1	Set 2	Set 3

Set 1	Set 2	Set 3

Set 1	Set 2	Set 3

FRIDAY

CORE EXERCISES

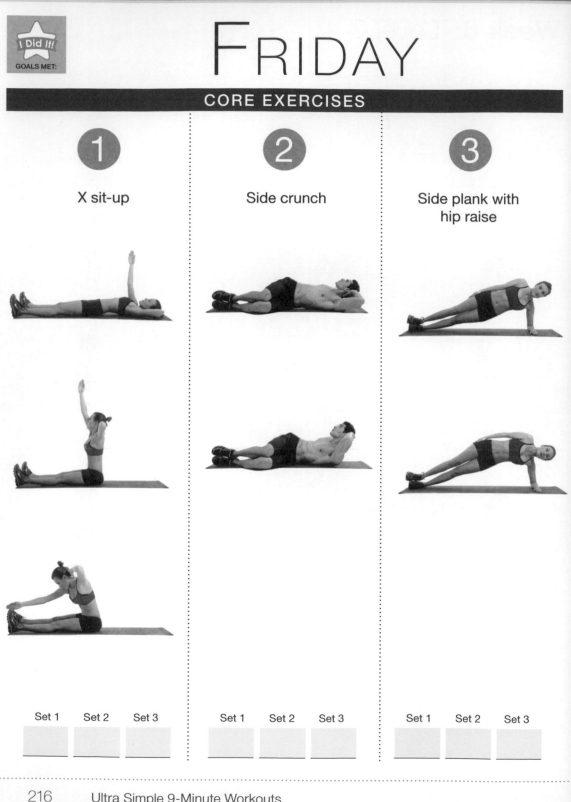

1

X sit-up

2

Side crunch

3

Side plank with
hip raise

Set 1   Set 2   Set 3

Set 1   Set 2   Set 3

Set 1   Set 2   Set 3

Week 6: Level 2

DATE:_____   WEIGHT:_____

LOWER BODY EXERCISES

1

Lunges with a twist

2

Clamshell with dumbbell

3

Side lunge

Set 1	Set 2	Set 3

Set 1	Set 2	Set 3

Set 1	Set 2	Set 3

I Did It!
GOALS MET:

SATURDAY

CARDIO EXERCISES

①	②	③
Front kick	Star jump	Uppercut

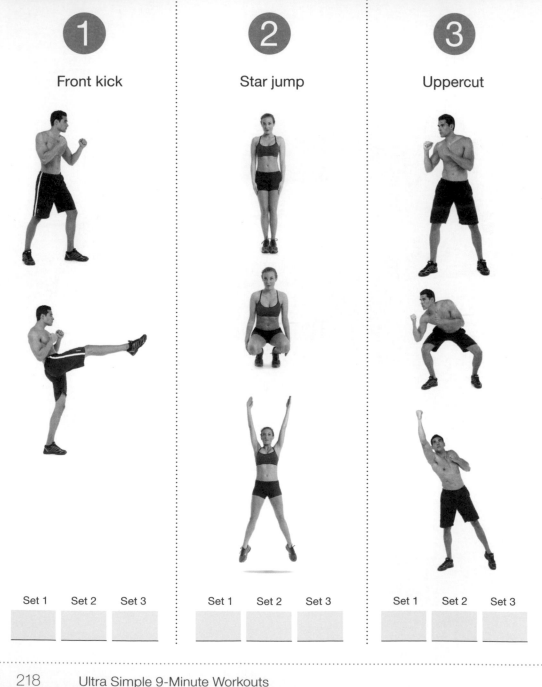

Set 1	Set 2	Set 3	Set 1	Set 2	Set 3	Set 1	Set 2	Set 3

Week 6: Level 2

DATE:_____   WEIGHT:_____

UPPER BODY EXERCISES

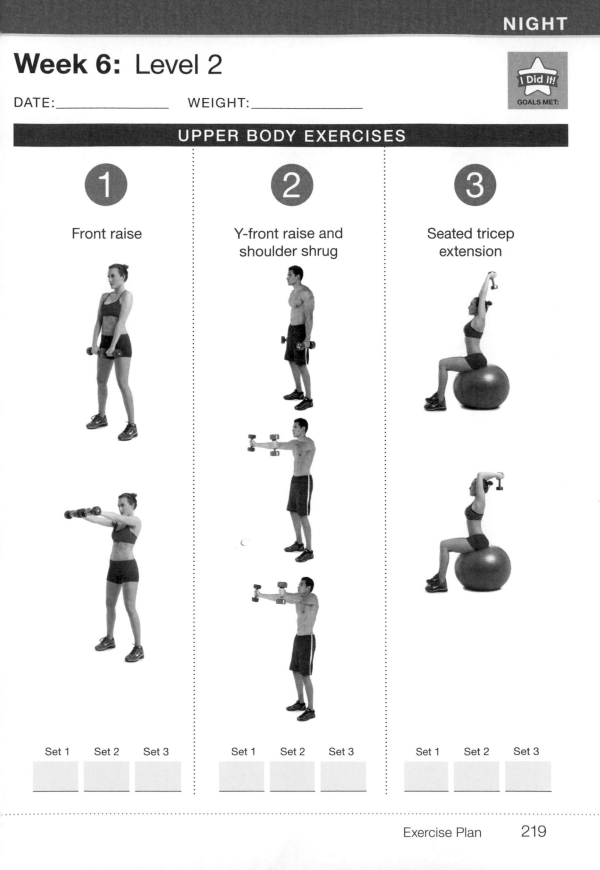

1

Front raise

2

Y-front raise and shoulder shrug

3

Seated tricep extension

Set 1	Set 2	Set 3

Set 1	Set 2	Set 3

Set 1	Set 2	Set 3

LOOKING BACK

DAYS I EXERCISED: WEEKLY ENERGY LEVEL:

Week 4: ☐ Mon. ☐ Tues. ☐ Wed. ☐ Thurs. ☐ Fri. ☐ Sat.   ☟ low   medium   high ☝

Week 5: ☐ Mon. ☐ Tues. ☐ Wed. ☐ Thurs. ☐ Fri. ☐ Sat.   ☟ low   medium   high ☝

Week 6: ☐ Mon. ☐ Tues. ☐ Wed. ☐ Thurs. ☐ Fri. ☐ Sat.   ☟ low   medium   high ☝

LEVEL 2 HIGHLIGHT

Your greatest moment from Level 2:

_____

_____

_____

_____

_____

_____

EXERCISE GOALS

Did you meet your Level 1 goals?

_____

_____

_____

_____

_____

_____

_____

IMPROVEMENTS

Ways to improve in the next level:

_____

_____

_____

_____

_____

_____

_____

_____

DATE:_____   WEIGHT:_____

LOOKING FORWARD

Your expectations for Level 3:

_____

_____

_____

_____

_____

_____

EXERCISE GOALS

Exercise goals for Level 3:

_____

_____

_____

_____

_____

_____

_____

NOTES

Obstacles, solutions, and thoughts on your progress:

_____

_____

_____

_____

_____

_____

_____

_____

MONDAY

CORE EXERCISES

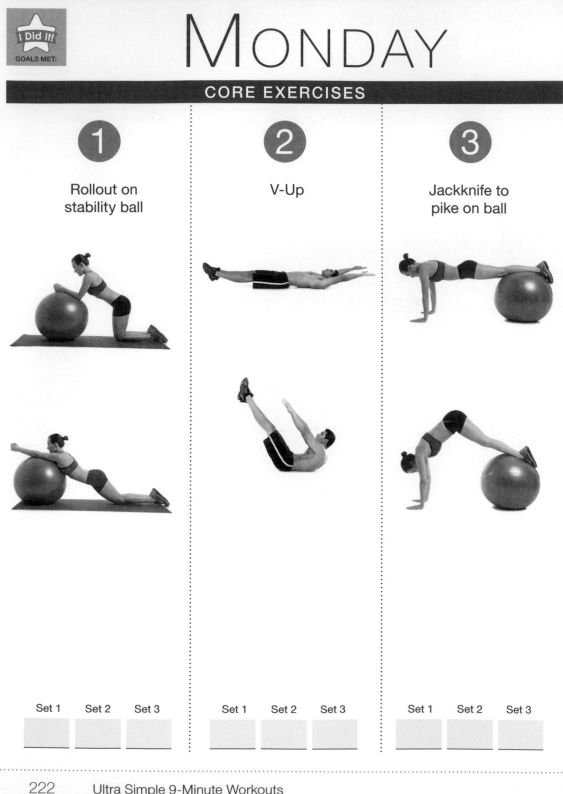

1

Rollout on stability ball

2

V-Up

3

Jackknife to pike on ball

Set 1	Set 2	Set 3

Set 1	Set 2	Set 3

Set 1	Set 2	Set 3

I Did It! GOALS MET:

Week 7: Level 3

DATE:_____ WEIGHT:_____

LOWER BODY EXERCISES

1

Squat kick

2

Sumo squats with dumbbell

3

Single leg dip

Set 1	Set 2	Set 3

Set 1	Set 2	Set 3

Set 1	Set 2	Set 3

I Did It!
GOALS MET:

TUESDAY

CARDIO EXERCISES

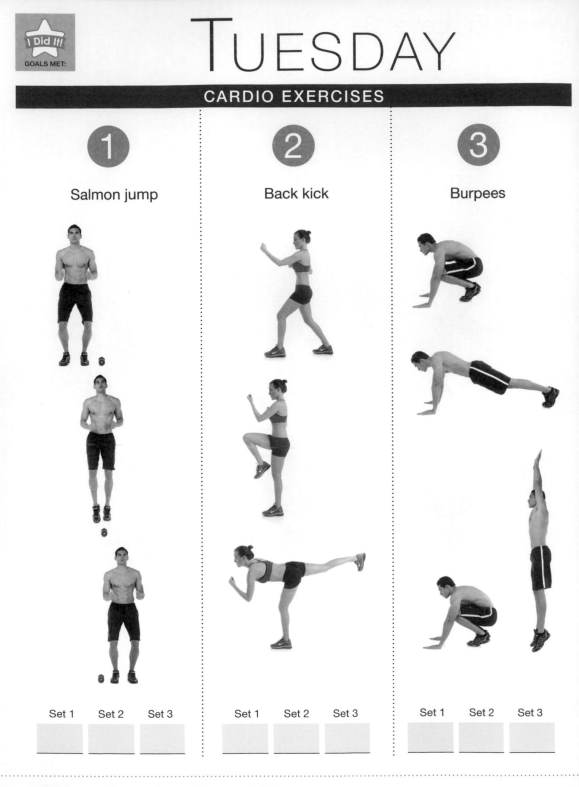

1 Salmon jump

2 Back kick

3 Burpees

Set 1	Set 2	Set 3

Set 1	Set 2	Set 3

Set 1	Set 2	Set 3

Week 7: Level 3

DATE:_____   WEIGHT:_____

UPPER BODY EXERCISES

1

Judo push-up

2

Dumbbell alternating shoulder press w/twist

3

Bicep curl to overhead press

Set 1	Set 2	Set 3

Set 1	Set 2	Set 3

Set 1	Set 2	Set 3

WEDNESDAY

CORE EXERCISES

1

2

3

Superman

Side plank with push-up

Russian twist with dumbbell

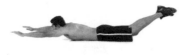
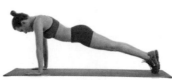
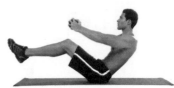

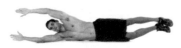
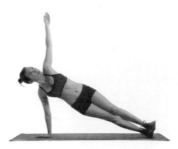
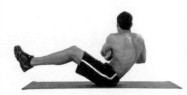

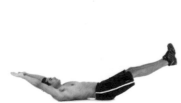
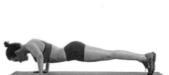
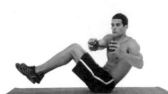
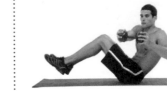

Set 1	Set 2	Set 3		Set 1	Set 2	Set 3		Set 1	Set 2	Set 3

Week 7: Level 3

DATE:_____   WEIGHT:_____

LOWER BODY EXERCISES

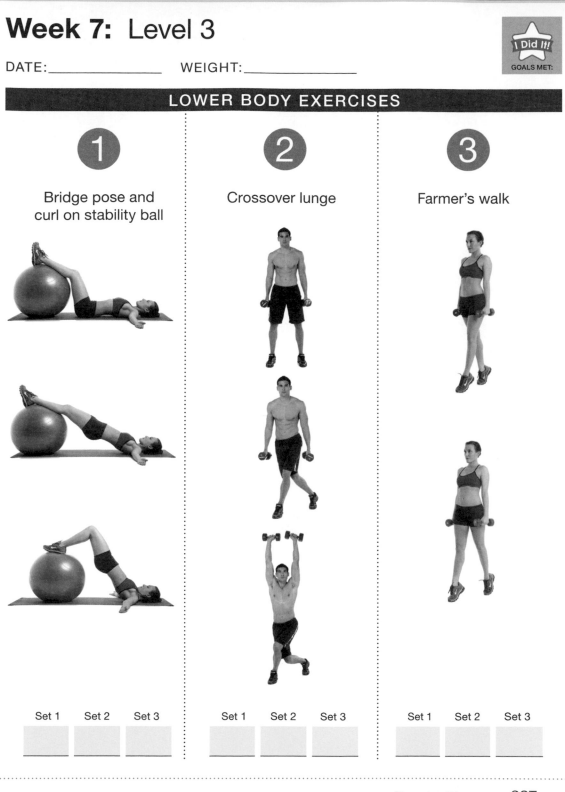

1 Bridge pose and curl on stability ball

2 Crossover lunge

3 Farmer's walk

Set 1	Set 2	Set 3

Set 1	Set 2	Set 3

Set 1	Set 2	Set 3

THURSDAY

CARDIO EXERCISES

1	**2**	**3**
Split jumps	Mountain climbers	Right-left punch

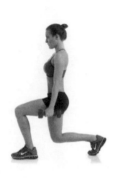
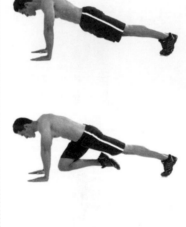
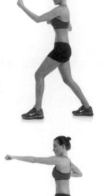

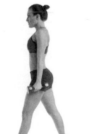
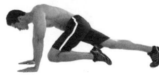
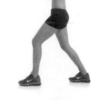

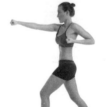

Set 1	Set 2	Set 3	Set 1	Set 2	Set 3	Set 1	Set 2	Set 3

Week 7: Level 3

DATE:_____   WEIGHT:_____

UPPER BODY EXERCISES

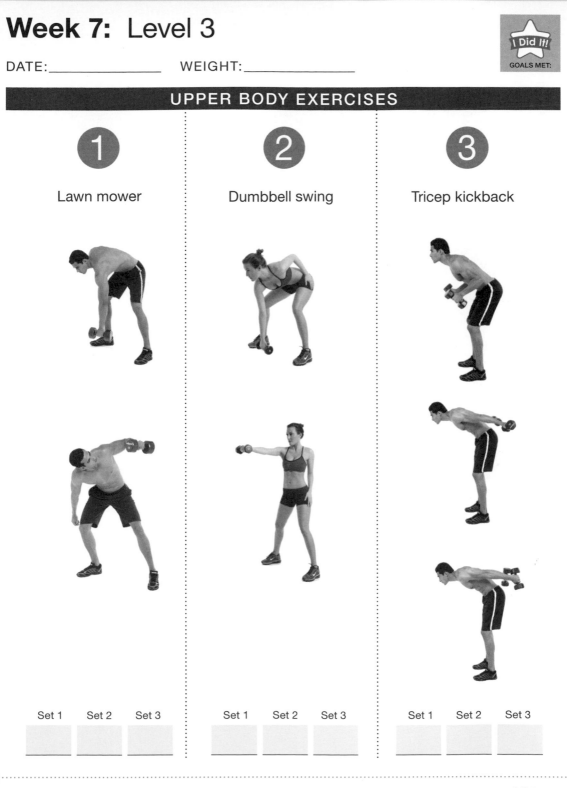

1

Lawn mower

2

Dumbbell swing

3

Tricep kickback

Set 1	Set 2	Set 3

Set 1	Set 2	Set 3

Set 1	Set 2	Set 3

I Did It!
GOALS MET:

FRIDAY

CORE EXERCISES

1	**2**	**3**
V-Up	Jackknife to pike on ball	Superman

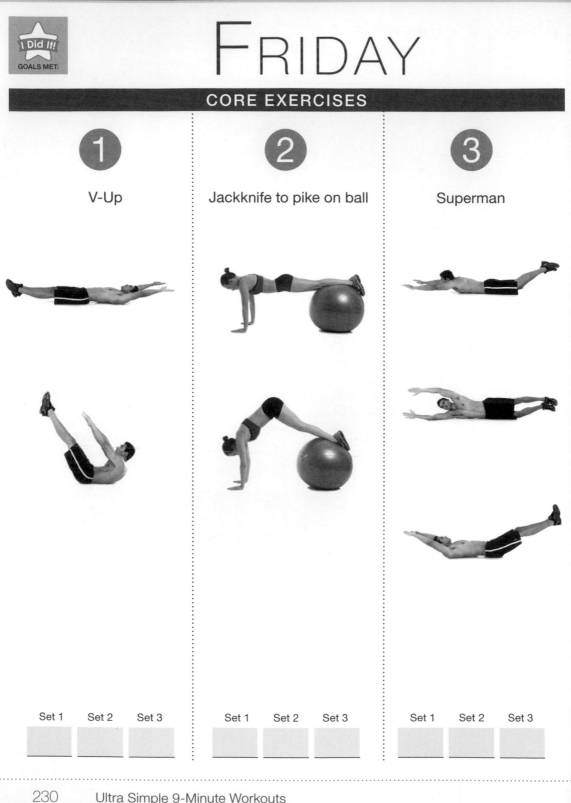

Set 1	Set 2	Set 3	Set 1	Set 2	Set 3	Set 1	Set 2	Set 3

Week 7: Level 3

DATE:_____   WEIGHT:_____

I Did It!
GOALS MET:

LOWER BODY EXERCISES

 1

Sumo squats with dumbbell

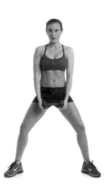

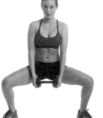

 2

Single leg dip

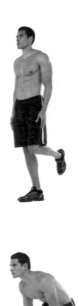

 3

Bridge pose and curl on stability ball

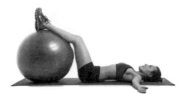

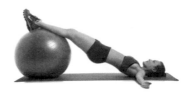

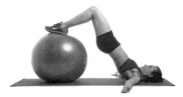

Set 1	Set 2	Set 3

Set 1	Set 2	Set 3

Set 1	Set 2	Set 3

I Did It!
GOALS MET:

SATURDAY

CORE EXERCISES

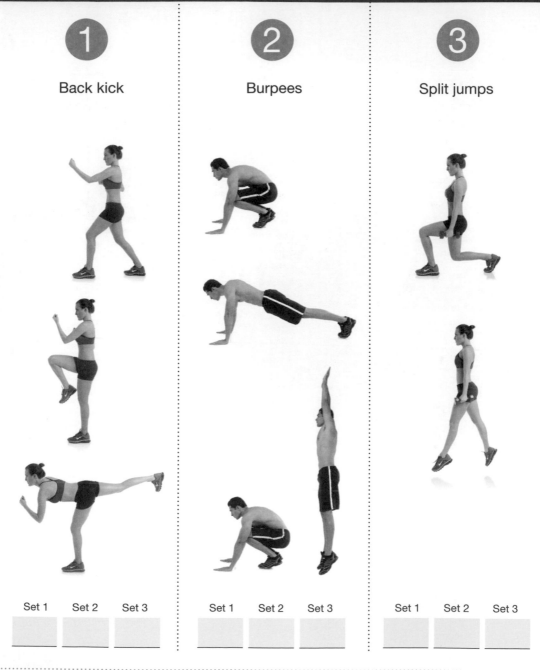

1	2	3
Back kick	Burpees	Split jumps

Set 1	Set 2	Set 3	Set 1	Set 2	Set 3	Set 1	Set 2	Set 3

Week 7: Level 3

DATE:_____   WEIGHT:_____

LOWER BODY EXERCISES

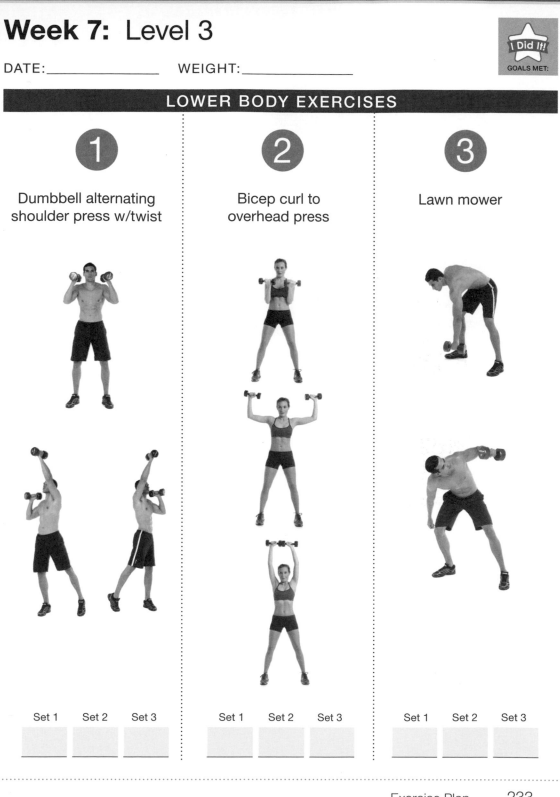

1

Dumbbell alternating
shoulder press w/twist

Set 1	Set 2	Set 3

2

Bicep curl to
overhead press

Set 1	Set 2	Set 3

3

Lawn mower

Set 1	Set 2	Set 3

I Did It! GOALS MET:

MONDAY

CORE EXERCISES

1	**2**	**3**
Side plank with push-up	Russian twist with dumbbell	Rollout on stability ball

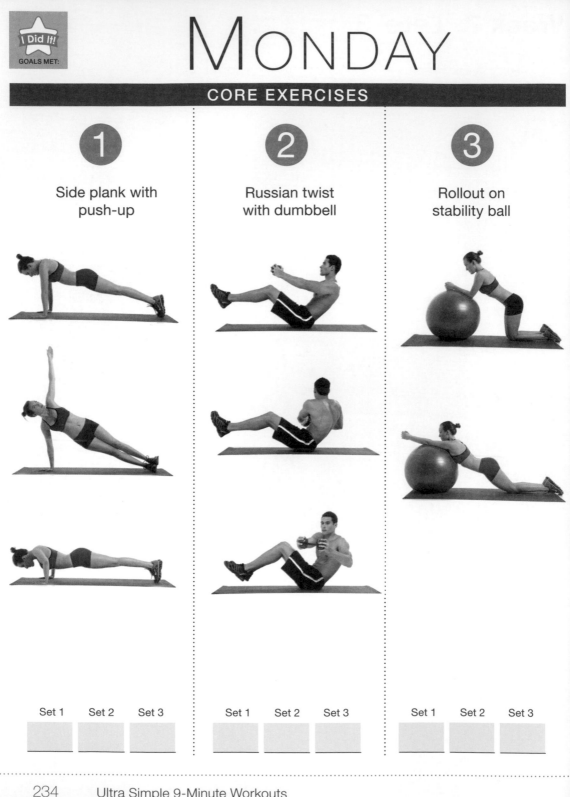

Set 1	Set 2	Set 3	Set 1	Set 2	Set 3	Set 1	Set 2	Set 3

Week 8: Level 3

DATE:_____ WEIGHT:_____

LOWER BODY EXERCISES

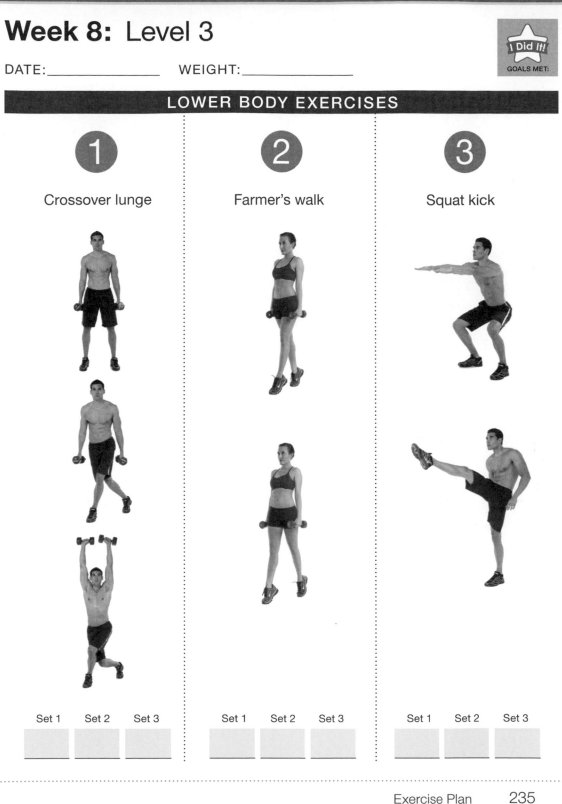

1 Crossover lunge

2 Farmer's walk

3 Squat kick

Set 1	Set 2	Set 3

Set 1	Set 2	Set 3

Set 1	Set 2	Set 3

TUESDAY

I Did It!
GOALS MET:

CARDIO EXERCISES

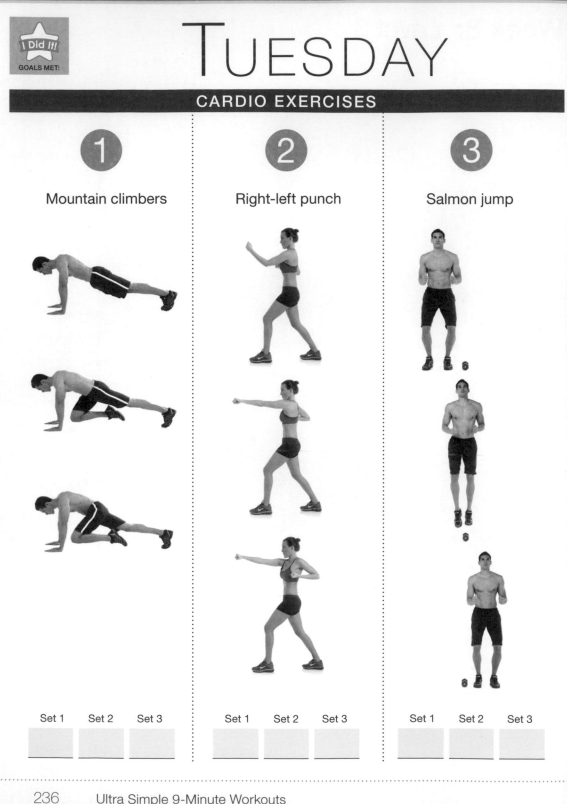

1 Mountain climbers

2 Right-left punch

3 Salmon jump

Set 1	Set 2	Set 3	Set 1	Set 2	Set 3	Set 1	Set 2	Set 3

Week 8: Level 3

DATE:_____   WEIGHT:_____

I Did It!
GOALS MET:

UPPER BODY EXERCISES

 1   **2**   **3**

Dumbbell swing   Tricep kickback   Judo push-up

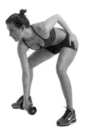
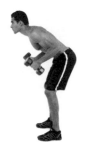
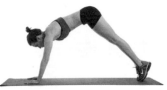

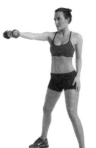
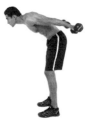
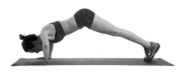

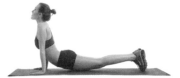

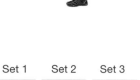
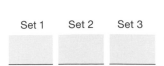

Set 1   Set 2   Set 3   Set 1   Set 2   Set 3   Set 1   Set 2   Set 3

WEDNESDAY

CORE EXERCISES

 1

Jackknife to pike on ball

 2

Superman

 3

Side plank with push-up

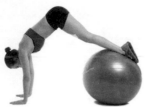

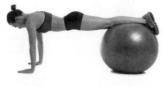

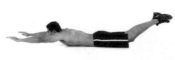

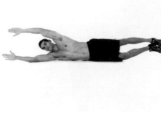

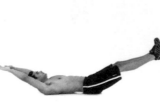

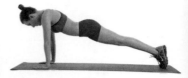

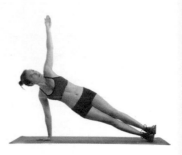

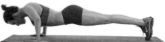

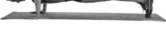

Set 1	Set 2	Set 3

Set 1	Set 2	Set 3

Set 1	Set 2	Set 3

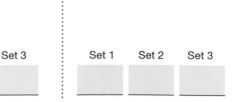

Week 8: Level 3

DATE:_____   WEIGHT:_____

LOWER BODY EXERCISES

1

Single leg dip

2

Bridge pose and curl on stability ball

3

Crossover lunge

Set 1	Set 2	Set 3

Set 1	Set 2	Set 3

Set 1	Set 2	Set 3

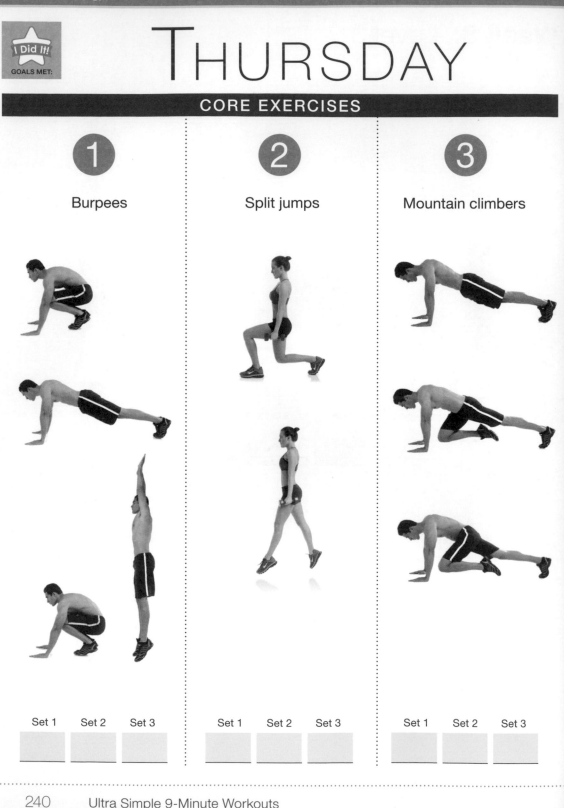

I Did It!
GOALS MET:

THURSDAY

CORE EXERCISES

1
Burpees

2
Split jumps

3
Mountain climbers

Set 1	Set 2	Set 3		Set 1	Set 2	Set 3		Set 1	Set 2	Set 3

Week 8: Level 3

DATE:_____ WEIGHT:_____

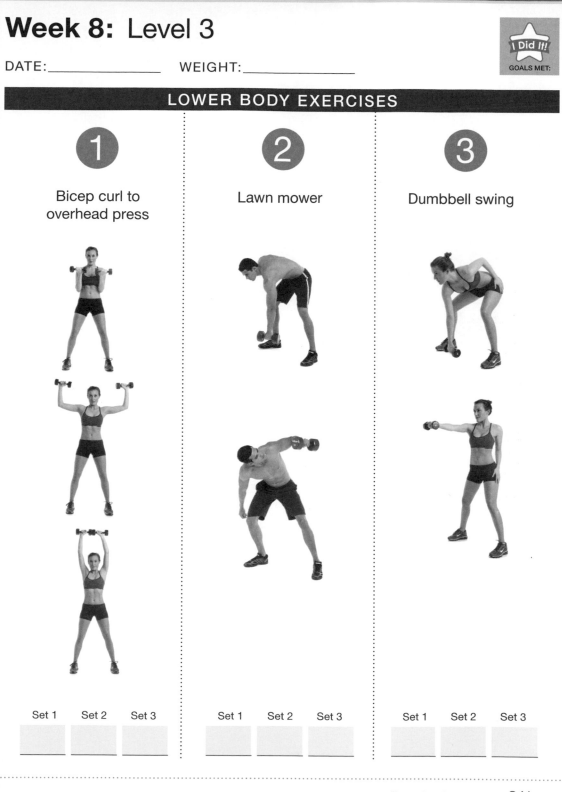

I Did It!
GOALS MET:

LOWER BODY EXERCISES

1
Bicep curl to overhead press

2
Lawn mower

3
Dumbbell swing

Set 1	Set 2	Set 3

Set 1	Set 2	Set 3

Set 1	Set 2	Set 3

FRIDAY

CORE EXERCISES

 1

 2

 3

Russian twist with dumbbell

Rollout on stability ball

V-Up

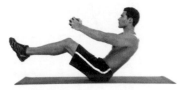

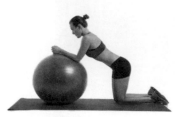

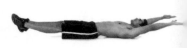

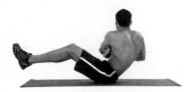

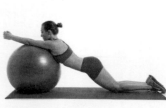

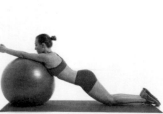

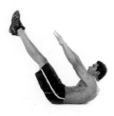

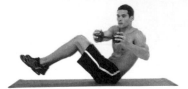

Set 1	Set 2	Set 3

Set 1	Set 2	Set 3

Set 1	Set 2	Set 3

Week 8: Level 3

DATE:_____   WEIGHT:_____

LOWER BODY EXERCISES

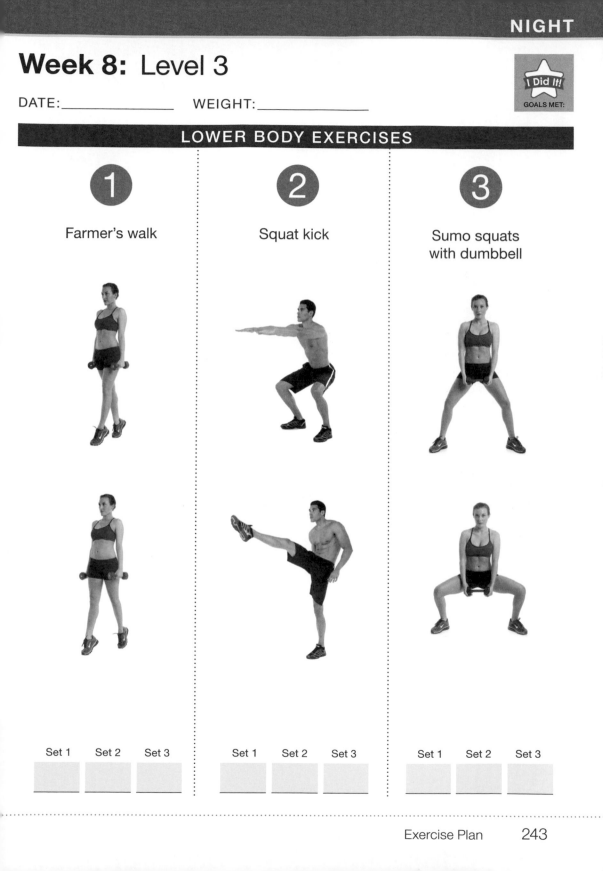

1

Farmer's walk

2

Squat kick

3

Sumo squats
with dumbbell

Set 1	Set 2	Set 3

Set 1	Set 2	Set 3

Set 1	Set 2	Set 3

I Did It!
GOALS MET:

SATURDAY

CARDIO EXERCISES

1	2	3
Right-left punch	Salmon jump	Back kick

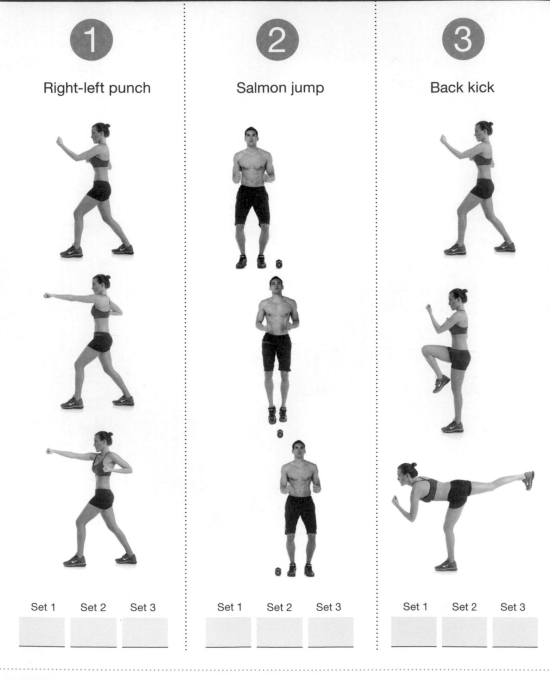

Set 1	Set 2	Set 3	Set 1	Set 2	Set 3	Set 1	Set 2	Set 3

Week 8: Level 3

DATE:_____ WEIGHT:_____

UPPER BODY EXERCISES

1

Tricep kickback

2

Judo push-up

3

Dumbbell alternating shoulder press w/twist

Set 1	Set 2	Set 3		Set 1	Set 2	Set 3		Set 1	Set 2	Set 3

I Did It!
GOALS MET:

MONDAY

CORE EXERCISES

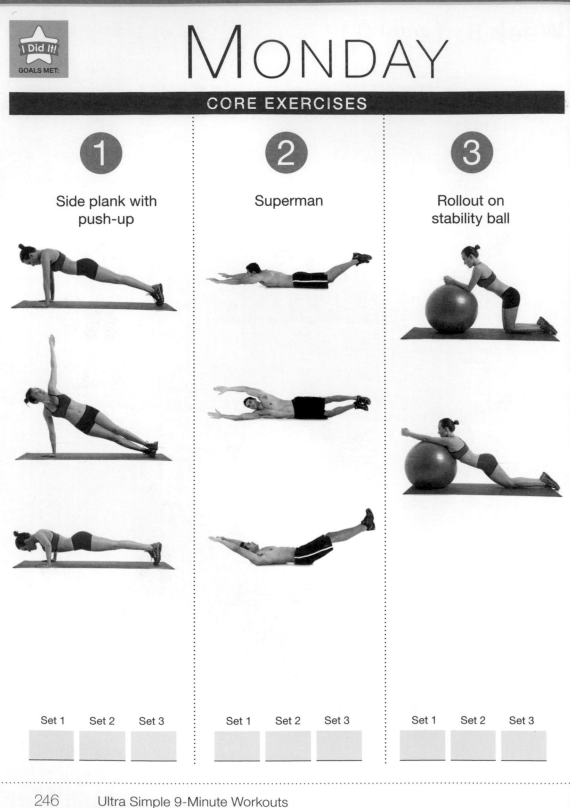

1

Side plank with push-up

2

Superman

3

Rollout on stability ball

Set 1   Set 2   Set 3

Set 1   Set 2   Set 3

Set 1   Set 2   Set 3

Week 9: Level 3

DATE:_____ WEIGHT:_____

I Did It!
GOALS MET:

LOWER BODY EXERCISES

1	**2**	**3**
Crossover lunge	Bridge pose and curl on stability ball	Squat kick

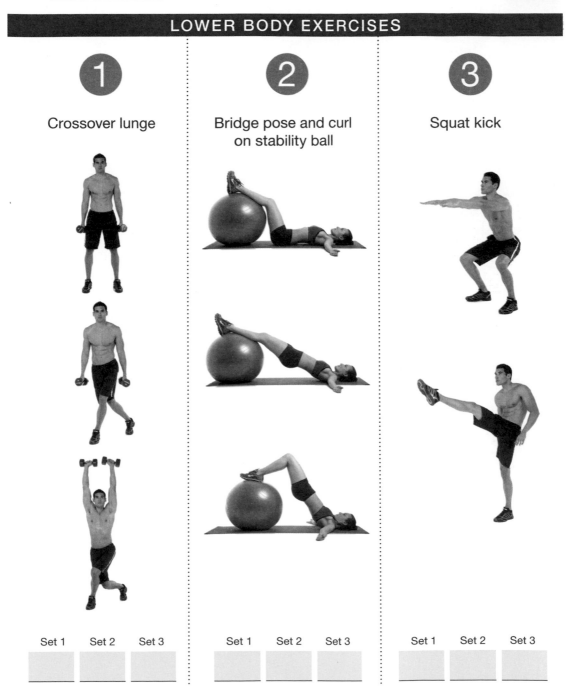

Set 1	Set 2	Set 3	Set 1	Set 2	Set 3	Set 1	Set 2	Set 3

TUESDAY

I Did It!
GOALS MET:

CORE EXERCISES

1	**2**	**3**
Mountain climbers	Split jumps	Salmon jump

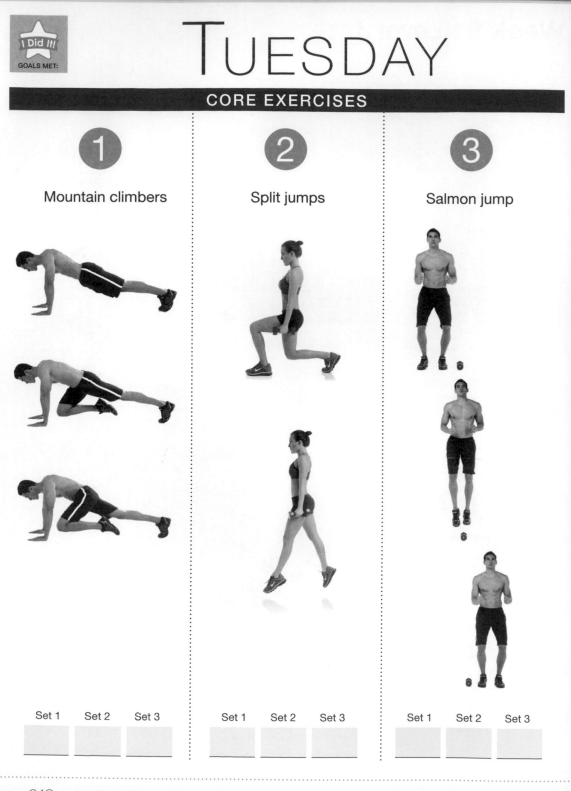

Set 1	Set 2	Set 3	Set 1	Set 2	Set 3	Set 1	Set 2	Set 3

Week 9: Level 3

DATE:_____   WEIGHT:_____

LOWER BODY EXERCISES

1

Dumbbell swing

2

Lawn mower

3

Judo push-up

Set 1	Set 2	Set 3

Set 1	Set 2	Set 3

Set 1	Set 2	Set 3

WEDNESDAY

CORE EXERCISES

 1

V-Up

 2

Jackknife to pike on ball

 3

Russian twist with dumbbell

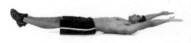

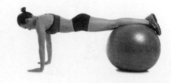

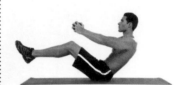

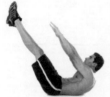

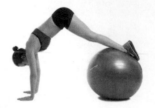

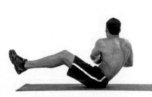

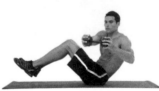

Set 1	Set 2	Set 3	Set 1	Set 2	Set 3	Set 1	Set 2	Set 3

Week 9: Level 3

DATE:_____ WEIGHT:_____

LOWER BODY EXERCISES

1

Sumo squats
with dumbbell

2

Single leg dip

3

Farmer's walk

Set 1	Set 2	Set 3

Set 1	Set 2	Set 3

Set 1	Set 2	Set 3

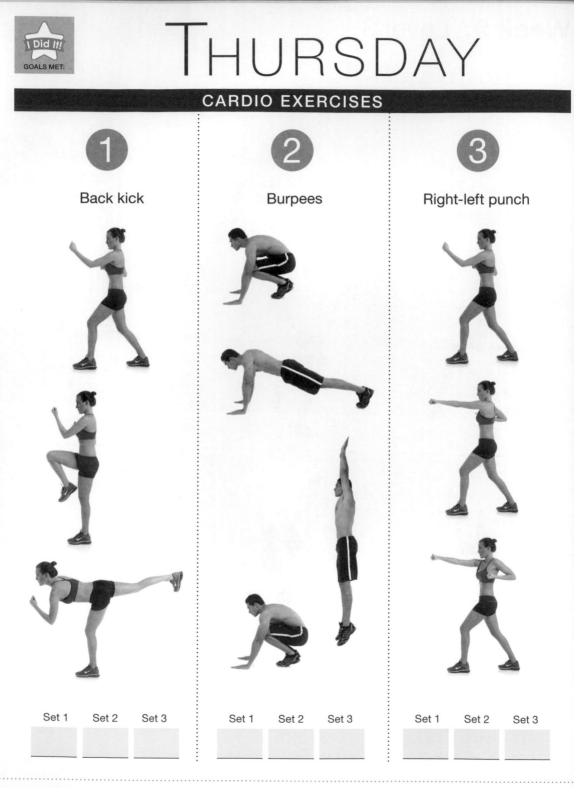

I Did It!
GOALS MET:

THURSDAY

CARDIO EXERCISES

1 Back kick

2 Burpees

3 Right-left punch

Set 1	Set 2	Set 3

Set 1	Set 2	Set 3

Set 1	Set 2	Set 3

Week 9: Level 3

DATE:_____   WEIGHT:_____

I Did It!
GOALS MET:

UPPER BODY EXERCISES

1

Dumbbell alternating shoulder press w/twist

2

Bicep curl to overhead press

3

Tricep kickback

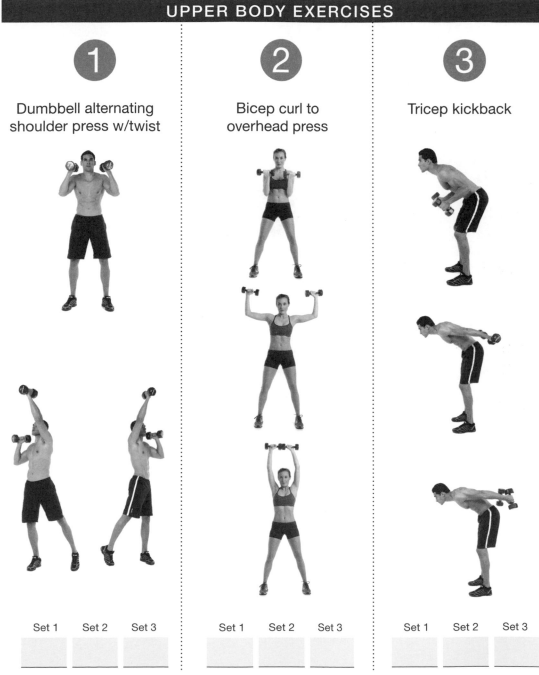

Set 1	Set 2	Set 3		Set 1	Set 2	Set 3		Set 1	Set 2	Set 3

I Did It!
GOALS MET:

FRIDAY

CORE EXERCISES

Rollout on stability ball

Russian twist with dumbbell

Side plank with push-up

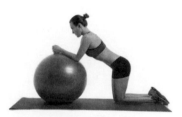

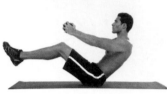

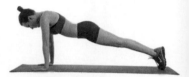

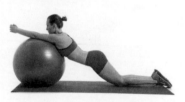

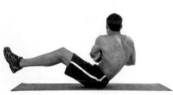

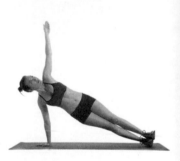

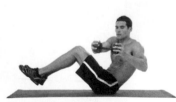

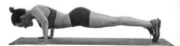

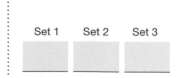

Set 1	Set 2	Set 3

Set 1	Set 2	Set 3

Set 1	Set 2	Set 3

Week 9: Level 3

DATE:_____ WEIGHT:_____

LOWER BODY EXERCISES

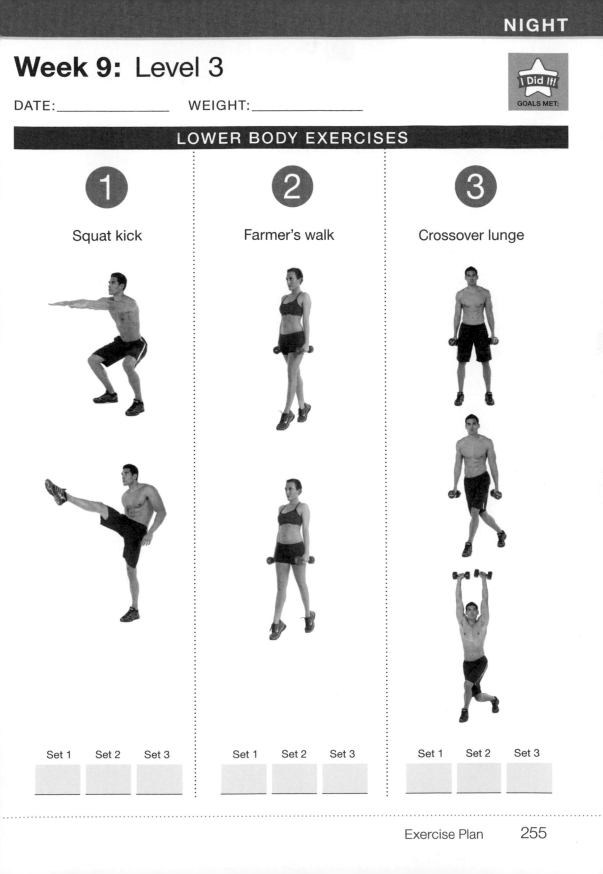

1 Squat kick

2 Farmer's walk

3 Crossover lunge

Set 1	Set 2	Set 3

Set 1	Set 2	Set 3

Set 1	Set 2	Set 3

I Did It!
GOALS MET:

SATURDAY

CARDIO EXERCISES

1	**2**	**3**
Salmon jump	Right-left punch	Mountain climbers

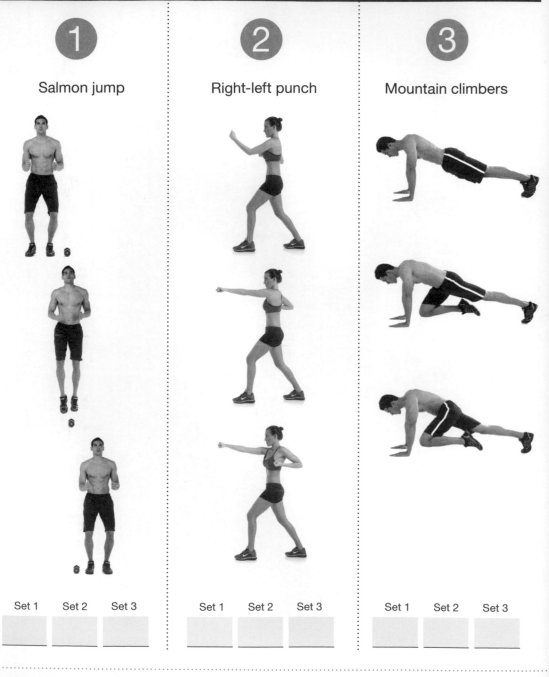

| Set 1 | Set 2 | Set 3 | | Set 1 | Set 2 | Set 3 | | Set 1 | Set 2 | Set 3 |

Week 9: Level 3

DATE:_____ WEIGHT:_____

I Did It!
GOALS MET:

UPPER BODY EXERCISES

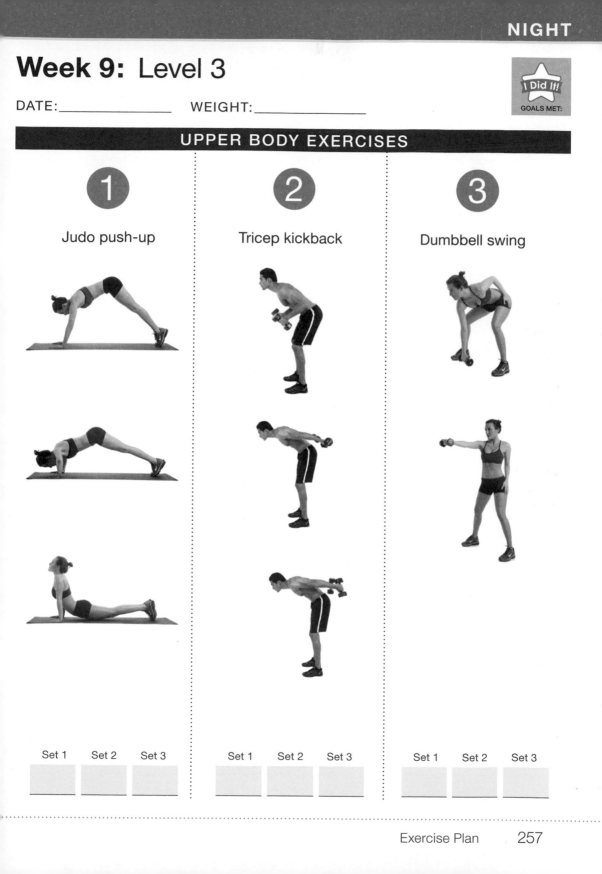

1   Judo push-up

2   Tricep kickback

3   Dumbbell swing

Set 1	Set 2	Set 3

Set 1	Set 2	Set 3

Set 1	Set 2	Set 3

DAYS I EXERCISED: **WEEKLY ENERGY LEVEL:**

Week 1: ☐ Mon. ☐ Tues. ☐ Wed. ☐ Thurs. ☐ Fri. ☐ Sat.   ♡ low   medium   high 👍

Week 2: ☐ Mon. ☐ Tues. ☐ Wed. ☐ Thurs. ☐ Fri. ☐ Sat.   ♡ low   medium   high 👍

Week 3: ☐ Mon. ☐ Tues. ☐ Wed. ☐ Thurs. ☐ Fri. ☐ Sat.   ♡ low   medium   high 👍

LEVEL 3 HIGHLIGHT

Your greatest moment from Level 3:

_____

_____

_____

_____

_____

_____

EXERCISE GOALS

Did you meet your Level 3 goals?

_____

_____

_____

_____

_____

_____

_____

IMPROVEMENTS

Ways to improve:

_____

_____

_____

_____

_____

_____

_____

_____

DATE:_____   WEIGHT:_____

LOOKING FORWARD

Your expectations for future fitness:

_____

_____

_____

_____

_____

_____

EXERCISE GOALS

Exercise goals after the program:

_____

_____

_____

_____

_____

_____

NOTES

Obstacles, solutions, and thoughts on your progress:

_____

_____

_____

_____

_____

_____

_____

_____

Notes

Maintaining Your Weight Loss

Congratulations, you made it through the program! What happens now? This chapter covers the ways to maintain your weight loss and to continue to lose even more weight — but first, you should celebrate your weight-loss accomplishments! Remember, use what you've learned in this book and celebrate without bingeing or indulging in a high-calorie meal. Healthy celebrations include going to a concert or sporting event, seeing a movie with a loved one, shopping for a new item of clothing to fit your slimmed-down shape, or treating yourself to a kitchen appliance you've had your eye on. If the reward helps you continue to lose weight, even better!

After you've sufficiently rewarded yourself for a job well done, it's time to think long-term. Do you want to continue losing weight with this diet and fitness program? Well, why not? If you followed the food and exercise tips, tricks, and secrets here you lost weight in a short amount of time without feeling stressed, starved, or deprived. And after a few weeks, these behaviors have had enough time to become real habits and lifestyle changes. So why stop now?

There are a few things to be aware of, however. For one, you may hit a point where your weight loss slows down from 1 or 2 pounds per week to less than 1 pound. You may even hit a plateau and stop losing weight all together. This is perfectly normal. Your body is slimming down, you have less weight and body fat to lose, and you are growing accustomed to eating less and exercising more. Consider getting a trainer who can help you mix up your routine, use new machines, and try new techniques you may never have considered. When you do the same exercises or strength training workout, you're firing the same muscle fibers again and again — and they begin to adapt. You may also need to work out longer to keep losing weight. But don't worry — as you build muscle and lose fat, your body will automatically burn more calories when it's at rest.

But truly, the greatest aspect you'll find about the *Ultra Simple 9-Minute Workouts* program is that exercising and eating right become a way of life! Plopping down on the couch with a bag of chips simply won't seem appealing to you anymore. And your body will have become used to eating smaller meals, so pigging out on half a pizza won't be on your mind.

Just don't lose your focus, stop watching your portion sizes, or get lazy with exercise. Read on for some great ways to enjoy your success but keep losing weight while sticking to your new, healthy lifestyle.

Start thinking of yourself as thin

Sadly, many people who slim down still view themselves as their former, fatter selves. They wear the same clothes they wore when they were heavier, or save a place in their closets for their "fat" clothes. Many overweight people shy away from wearing bright colors that draw attention to problem areas, and still end up dressing in all black after they lose weight. But now is the time to embrace change and show off your hard work! Invest in a few new pieces and feel proud wearing them. Not only are you rewarding yourself, you'll look better too. Wearing clothing that is too big for you isn't flattering and will only hide your flatter stomach and more defined arms and legs. And why not start some closet spring cleaning? Anything dowdy, oversized, or out of shape can be donated to charity. Some people hold on to all their old clothes because they're afraid they'll gain the weight back, but getting rid of them means you're saying goodbye to the old you who sat on the couch with a bowl of ice cream every night. This new you exercises, eats right throughout the week, and celebrates a healthy, thinner figure. Just don't go on a shopping spree if you're planning to lose more weight (and you should be!). Wait until you're down 2 full sizes to splurge on a new wardrobe.

Revamp your daily routine to include fitness

So how many days a week are you going to need to exercise to maintain or increase your weight loss after you've completed this program? Consider that the men and women of the National Weight Control Registry (a roster of more than 6,000 participants who, on average, have lost 66 pounds and kept them off for five and a half years), report exercising for an average of 60 to 75 minutes daily. If you are not the type of person who enjoys going to a gym you'll need to integrate other forms of calorie-burning activities into your life. For instance, vacuuming for an hour burns 220 calories, grocery shopping requires 180 calories, and an afternoon of gardening, sweeping, and raking leaves expends 270 calories. If your home or office has stairs, walking up them in a moderate manner for 15 minutes burns 120 calories. Need a room in your house painted? Do it yourself and burn 340 calories an hour. Live in an area with snow? You've hit the jackpot — shoveling snow for an hour burns 600 calories. Combining a few of these forms of aerobic activity is the equivalent of spending a couple of hours at the gym.

Make new friends who also care about healthy living

If you've joined a gym or fitness class or group, you have ample opportunities to make new friends, and the best part is, these are people who care about being healthy and staying slim. Losing weight also opens doors to more confidence, and many times, a new social life. Accept more invitations to parties and get-togethers; wear something that makes you feel amazing and that shows off your hard work. Being around people who share your interest in eating well and being healthy, as well as people who praise your weight loss, will keep you motivated to keep working hard.

Must have a treat? Keep it reasonable

If you really want to enjoy a treat in the form of food, keep it under 250 calories. A small sundae or miniature cupcake will do the trick. Just consciously remind yourself that this is a treat at the end of your hard work, and not an invitation to go back to your old bad habits. This is a one-time celebration and not a weekly event.

Beat the weight-loss plateau

Naturally, the same diet and workout aren't going to produce the same results week after week. There are many ways to break through the plateaus you'll inevitably encounter. Let's say you have been doing cardio 5 days a week for 45 minutes; either add an extra 15 minutes to a few workouts, or else turn a normal session into an interval session just by interspersing 30 to 60-second bursts of speed and intensity every few minutes. Or break through a plateau by changing up your meal routine. For instance, try eating a bigger lunch with more fiber and a smaller dinner. This can help take advantage of when your metabolism is faster during the day.

Document your progress with photos and measurements

The scale may not always accurately reflect your weight loss, considering that muscle greatly outweighs fat, and water weight can be a factor as well. The best way to document your progress is with photos (take them in a similar swimsuit each time) and by measuring yourself around the hips, thighs, stomach, chest, and arms. Losing inches (along with pant and dress sizes) are the true test of your weight-loss success. And, seeing your new, slimmer self reflected in photos is one of the best testaments to how well this program has worked for you. When you feel like giving up or going back to your old ways, you can look at your Before and After photos, and feel fantastic about how far you've come and how much weight you've lost all over. This confidence and pride are what keeps you going.

Stave off boredom

One common excuse for abandoning a workout or weight-loss program is boredom. Naturally, people get sick of the same gym grind or meal plan. When boredom starts to threaten your weight loss, it's time to introduce a new form of exercise or try one that never gets dull. Yoga, for instance, is a fantastic full-body workout and is a practice that is ever-evolving. Because there's always a new level of intensity or difficulty to reach, your body will never get complacent, and you won't get bored. Or try taking up something that takes a long time to master, such as surfing, which is a great full-body workout — and fun too!

The same concept goes for the foods you eat. Although a minority of people say they like the routine of eating the same thing at every meal, most people get bored and eventually succumb to cravings. Change up your go-to low-calorie meals in easy ways. Swap grilled salmon for chicken in a salad; add shredded chicken and avocado to a bowl of soup; experiment with a new vegetable on the side of your dinner.

Update your music playlist every month

Music inspires you to get moving and keep moving. A great playlist keeps your energy up, but, just like anything, you will get bored if you're listening to the same songs day in and day out. It's a great idea to make separate playlists for different workouts of varying intensities. For example, a super-fast set of songs for running, interval training, and weight lifting, a slower set for jogging, and a relaxing, calming set for stretching and cooling down. Try varying the songs on each playlist every month. Check on your local radio stations' websites for what's new, or visit ShapeMagazine.com — they offer great monthly playlists for up-tempo workouts, and you can click right through to purchase the songs on iTunes.

Calculate your new daily calorie allowance

Now that you've lost weight, you may be ready to simply maintain your weight, or, you may be interested in losing even more. To do that, you need to calculate your new BMR (it changes as you lose weight) and new daily calorie allowance. That is the number of calories you'd need to eat each day to maintain your current weight. If you want to lose more weight, you should create another Calorie Deficit, in the same way you did throughout this program.

The following equation uses your new BMR and factors in activity level:

To calculate your new BMR:

Women BMR = 655 + (4.3 x weight in pounds) + (4.7 x height in inches) - (4.7 x age in years)

Men BMR = 66 + (6.3 x weight in pounds) + (12.9 x height in inches) - (6.8 x age in years)

To find daily calorie allowance, choose the appropriate activity level, and multiply your BMR accordingly.

Sedentary (little or no exercise):

Calorie-Calculation = BMR x 1.2

Lightly active (light exercise/activity 1-3 days/week):

Calorie-Calculation = BMR x 1.375

Moderately active (moderate exercise/activity 3-5 days/week):

Calorie-Calculation = BMR x 1.55

Very active (hard exercise/activity 6-7 days a week):

Calorie-Calculation = BMR x 1.725

Extra active (very hard exercise/activity, physical job, or sports conditioning):

Calorie-Calculation = BMR x 1.9

The result of this calculation is the number of calories you can eat every day to maintain your current weight. If you want to lose more weight, reduce your calories to a number below your maintenance level. Just keep in mind that, according to the American College of Sports Medicine, calorie intake should never drop below 1200 calories per day for women or 1800 calories per day for men. Even those amounts are incredibly low. Keep your calories at a level that allows you to feel full and gives you enough energy for exercise.

Do what works for others

An important part of observing National Weight Control Registry members is determining how they manage to keep the weight off when such a huge majority of dieters fail to do so. In the end, there are 3 main factors that members continue to report again and again, which this book has already highlighted. Stick with these moving forward and you're sure to keep the weight off and lose even more. In order to maintain their weight loss, NWCR members:

- 78% eat breakfast every day
- 62% watch less than 10 hours of TV per week
- 90% exercise, on average, about 1 hour per day

Get your family and friends involved in your new lifestyle

The only way to maintain this new, healthier way of life is to get the people closest to you onboard as well. That means being active with your family and friends. If you have kids, take up an activity that you can all do together, such as horseback riding, skiing, cycling, surfing, or even yoga. If you have very young children, a game of tag is enough to get you all active and moving together.

Invite your friends to be active with you as well. Most people will be excited and willing to try a new activity with you, especially if they have witnessed your weight-loss success firsthand.

Your family and friends should also join you in your efforts to eat low-calorie, low-fat meals as often as possible. Try adding shredded vegetables, such as carrots, squash, or zucchini, into pasta sauces or substituting meatless products into burritos and omelets — your fellow diners will never know the difference! Serve healthy desserts, such as fresh fruit with low-fat whipped topping, and your family will start to crave the same healthy foods that are helping you lose weight.

Tell Us Your Success Story!

Did you lose weight, break bad habits, and make new healthy ones with this book? We love when our readers share their weight-loss success stories with us!

Please tell us your story, your initial weight and measurements, your expectations for this diet and fitness program, etc. Tell us what you liked or didn't like about this book, and what you found useful or wished we had included. Also, tell us how you feel with your new slimmer and healthier body. Or maybe you want to share your best advice for others who are struggling with their weight.

Please include the following information:

- Your name:
- Phone number:
- E-mail:
- Your story!
- Before and After photos, if possible

Please email this information to info@WSPublishingGroup.com or send a letter to WS Publishing Group, 15373 Innovation Drive, Suite 360; San Diego, CA 92128.

Notes

Ultra Simple 9-Minute Workouts

Interval Timer
Workout & Fitness PRO

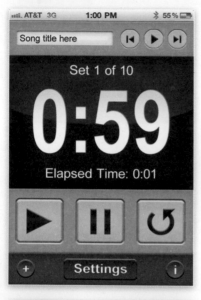

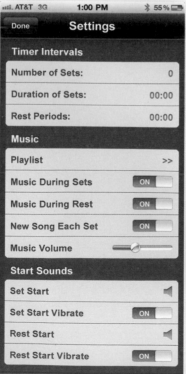

Working out has never been easier!
The *Interval Timer: Workout & Fitness PRO* keeps you motivated and makes exercise fun.

Special Features:
- Large, easy-to-read display & buttons
- Tracks number of sets performed
- Shows elapsed time and rest periods
- Gives multiple cue options for sets and rest periods
- Plays music from your iTunes library

So easy to use:
1) Enter the number of sets you desire, as well as the length of time for each set and rest period.

2) Select a custom ringtone or set your iPhone to vibrate to cue you at the start of each set and/or rest period.

Or, play your favorite music from your iTunes Library. You can even choose a new song to start off each set!